ADVANCES IN THE BIOSCIENCES

Volume 72

SMALL CELL LUNG CANCER

ADVANCES IN THE BIOSCIENCES

Latest volumes in the series:

SMALL CELL LUNG CANCER

Proceedings of the International Conference
on Small Cell Lung Cancer
27–28 March 1987, Ravenna, Italy

Editors:

M. MARANGOLO

and

G. FIORENTINI

Oncologia Medica, Ospedale Civile, Ravenna, Italy

PERGAMON PRESS · OXFORD · NEW YORK
BEIJING · FRANKFURT · SÃO   PAULO · SYDNEY · TOKYO · TORONTO

U.K.	Pergamon Press plc, Headington Hill Hall, Oxford OX3 0BW, England
U.S.A.	Pergamon Press, Inc., Maxwell House, Fairview Park, Elmsford, New York 10523, U.S.A.
PEOPLE'S REPUBLIC OF CHINA	Pergamon Press, Room 4037, Qianmen Hotel, Beijing, People's Republic of China
FEDERAL REPUBLIC OF GERMANY	Pergamon Press GmbH, Hammerweg 6, D-6242 Kronberg, Federal Republic of Germany
BRAZIL	Pergamon Editora Ltda, Rua Eça de Queiros, 346, CEP 04011, Paraiso, São Paulo, Brazil
AUSTRALIA	Pergamon Press Australia Pty Ltd., P.O. Box 544, Potts Point, N.S.W. 2011, Australia
JAPAN	Pergamon Press, 5th Floor, Matsuoka Central Building, 1-7-1 Nishishinjuku, Shinjuku-ku, Tokyo 160, Japan
CANADA	Pergamon Press Canada Ltd., Suite No. 271, 253 College Street, Toronto, Ontario, Canada M5T 1R5

First edition 1988

ISBN: 0–08–036631–7

ISSN: 0065–3446

In order to make this volume available as economically and as rapidly as possible the authors' typescripts have been reproduced in their original forms. This method unfortunately has its typographical limitations but it is hoped that they in no way distract the reader.

Printed in Great Britain by A. Wheaton & Co. Ltd., Exeter

Contents

Contents

Increasing Incidence and Mortality Rate of Small Cell Lung Cancer: an Emerging Problem?

M. Geddes and E. Chellini

Epidemiology Unit, Center for Study and Cancer
Prevention, Florence, Italy

ABSTRACT

The paper describes mortality trends for Lung Cancer in Italy, recent mortality rates in comparison with other Countries and incidence rates by sex in some Italian areas. The frequency of Small Cell Cancer of the Lung (SCCL) is reported from European and non European population based and hospital based studies. Methodologic problems in evaluating temporal trends by histologic type are overviewed. Specific risk factors and survival rates for SCCL are summarized. In conclusion, while an increase in incidence and mortality rates from SCCL is hypothized together with the increase in incidence and mortality from Lung Cancer as a whole, there is no evidence of an increase in the relative importance of this histologic type in comparison to other types of Lung Cancer.

KEYWORDS

Lung cancer, histologic types, small cell, incidence, mortality, trend.

INTRODUCTION

Are the small cell lung cancer (SCCL) incidence and mortality rates increasing? There is no univocal answer to this question. In Italy mortality rates for lung cancer as a whole have shown a striking increase in the last decades: if it is assumed that the proportion of SCCL has been stable during this period compared to the other histological types, this means that a relevant increase in small cell cancer absolute numbers has occurred both in males and in females. Last year (1986) about 26,000 people died from lung cancer in Italy: therefore about 5,000 deaths out of these 26,000 have to be considered as caused by SCCL. These figures emphasise the importance of this specific pathology. The attention given by researchers to this specific histologic type of lung cancer is due not only to its therapeutical problems but also to the relationship it seems to have with specific risk factors, which seem to be involved in the overall increase of lung cancer in the population.

However, temporal trends of incidence rates by specific site have to

be interpreted with caution, because of the variability over time of
diagnostic procedures, classification criteria, access of the popula
tion to the health services, etc.;   these biases become even more
relevant in evaluating incidence trends by histological type, and a
review of the available data at an international level does not point
out nor exclude clearly a relative increase over time of SCCL in com
parison to the other histological types.
The following is an overview on lung cancer descriptive epidemiology
in Italy in recent years focussed particularly on SCCL, compared with
other main histologic types.

LUNG CANCER MORTALITY IN ITALY

Lung cancer has been the main cause of death from cancer in Italy sin
ce 1974 (Capocaccia, 1984). Mortality rates continue to increase (Ta
ble 1) both in males and in females, contrary to the situation in re
cent years in several other industrialized countries including the U-
nited States (Horm, 1986) and Great Britain (Doll, 1982).

TABLE 1 Lung Cancer:Mortality Stand.Rates x100,000
Inh. (Standard: Italian Population 1971) from 1970
to 1981.   Age 0-74

| Year | Rate | |
	Males	Females
1970	42.2	5.7
1971	44.7	5.5
1972	45.9	5.9
1973	47.3	6.2
1974	49.1	6.2
1975	50.9	6.4
1976	53.0	6.7
1977	54.5	7.0
1978	56.1	6.7
1979	57.9	7.2
1980	60.5	7.2
1981	60.0	7.5

(Capocaccia, 1984, 1985, 1986)

Mortality from this pathology shows, in our country, notable differen
ces among territories, with higher mortality in the Nort-East and a
progressive decrease towards the South of Italy (Table 2).

Lung cancer mortality rates in Italy are average to high, particularly
for males, compared with other industrialized countries (Table 3).

TABLE 2 Lung Cancer:Mortality Stand.Rates x100,000 inh. (Standard: Italian Population 1971) in 1981 in Different Parts of Italy. Age 0-74.(Capocaccia,1984)

Area	Rate	
	Males	Females
North	72.4	8.9
Center	57.6	7.7
South	43.3	5.0

TABLE 3 Lung Cancer: Mortality Standardized Rates x 100,000 inh. (Standard: World Population) in 1983 All Ages

Males		Females	
Country	Rate	Country	Rate
Hungary	67.2	Hong Kong	23.9
England	65.8	USA	19.9
Canada	56.9	England	19.4
USA	56.8	Singapore	19.1
Italy **	55.9	Canada	16.9
Hong Kong	54.6	Cuba	14.5
Singapore	54.3	New Zealand	13.7
Uruguay **	53.8	Hungary	11.3
New Zealand	51.5	Australia	11.0
F.R.G.	48.7	Sweden	8.3
Australia	46.4	Japan	7.7
France	44.2	Israel	7.5
Cuba	39.3	F.R.G.	6.7
Japan	27.5	Italy **	6.3
Sweden	24.9	Mexico	4.7
Israel	23.0	France	4.1
Mexico	13.0	Uruguay **	4.1
Perù	7.7	Perù	2.6
Egypt *	2.6	Egypt *	1.0
SriLanka	1.6	SriLanka	0.8

* 1980
** 1982

Of particular relevance are age-specific rates in males which place Italy third for the age-groups 35-44 and 45-54 (Table 4). We consider these last rates to be a fair indication of what we might expect in future decades when these generations reach an age at which lung cancer is more frequent. This is an alarming phenomenon as it leads us to suppose that the present increase in lung cancer mortality will continue. It should be considered that it was only after the second world war, that smoking habits in Italy increased; therefore it is only in relatively recent years that cancer mortality rates have reached those apparent 20 years ago in other industrialized countries.

Another aspect to be considered is the increase, in recent years, in lung cancer mortality in females. In 1985 in the United States, (Cancer Statistics, 1985) lung cancer became the main cause of death from cancer in females. If the smoking habits of Italian women continue to increase, we can expect a similar phenomenon within the next 20-30 years.

TABLE 4 Lung Cancer: Mortality Standardized Rates x 100,000 inh. (Standard: World Population) in 1981 in Males   Age   35-44 and 45-54.

35-44 years		45-54 years	
Country	Rate	Country	Rate
Uruguay**	19.5	Hungary	87.7
Hungary	18.3	Uruguay **	84.8
Italy **	12.0	Italy * *	80.2
USA	11.8	USA	76.4
France	11.7	France	65.4
Honk Kong	10.1	Hong Kong	59.8
F.R.G.	10.0	England	59.4
New Zealand	9.8	New Zealand	58.3
Canada	8.7	Canada	57.3
Singapore	7.9	Australia	51.7
Cuba	7.9	F.R.G.	51.0
England	7.6	Singapore	47.2
Australia	7.4	Cuba	34.4
Sweden	4.2	Sweden	24.9
Israel	3.8	Israel	24.8
Japan	3.6	Japan	18.1
Mexico	2.1	Mexico	13.0
Egypt *	2.0	Perù	7.8
Perù	0.9	Egypt *	6.0

* 1980   ** 1982

LUNG CANCER INCIDENCE

The increase in lung cancer incidence rates is evident from data provided by the old-established Cancer Registries such as the Cancer Registries of the Scandinavian Countries (Kvale, 1982) and Cancer Registries of the USA (Dodds, 1986) etc.

As far as Italy is concerned, national rates are not available; only incidence rates relating to the areas to which currently active Cancer Registries are referred are available. Table 5 shows incidence rates by sex, standardized according to European and World populations, of some Italian Cancer Registries and of other European Countries.

In Italy only the Varese Cancer Registry has provided data for two successive periods showing, also in this case, an increase through time in lung cancer incidence.

TABLE 5   Standardized Incidence Rates of Lung Cancer
in Some Italian Areas by Sex and Comparison with
some other European Registries (Standard: European
and World Population).   All Ages

Cancer Registry	Years of observ.	Males Europ. pop.	World pop.	Females Europ. pop.	World pop.
Varese	1976-77	100.9	70.4	8.3	5.8
Varese	1978-81	117.5	80.9	9.0	6.1
Trieste	1984	124.3	82.6	25.0	16.7
Parma	1978-82	79.1	56.1	9.8	6.9
Firenze	1984	82.1	57.4	8.6	5.9
Latina	1982-85	62.5	43.1	5.8	4.1
Ragusa	1981-84	54.8	37.4	5.1	3.4
Birmingham	1973-76	-	79.8	-	13.7
Sweden	1983	-	25.4	-	8.9
Denmark	1982	-	56.5	-	18.5
Geneva	1978-82	104.7	72.2	14.7	10.3
Vaud	1979-83	85.3	59.2	10.7	7.3

As regards age at lung cancer onset or diagnosis, several studies
(Geddes, 1984; Klaassen, 1986) show differences between the two sexes.
Age at onset is younger in the female sex, in spite of more   restricted smoking habits and lower exposure to occupational risk
factors. This has resulted in a hypothesis on the action of predispos
ing endogenous factors in female sex (Klaassen, 1986) - factors which
have yet to be evaluated.

FREQUENCY OF MAIN HISTOLOGIC TYPES

Comparing the frequency of various histologic types, expecially SCCL,
in different series, poses several interpretative problems, notably:
a- The interpretation of histologic evidence even if it uses identical classification (e.g., the W.H.O. classification) is anyway proble
matic. Some data in this regard are quite comforting (Hanai, 1987;
Yesner, 1973), showing for SCCL a good concordance among various pathologists. Probably, however, concordance is less good among pathologists of different schools or with different experience.
b- Histologic   types have a different frequency in males and females;
therefore a separate comparison between the two sexes is appropriate
(Greenberg, 1984).
c- There are consistent percentage differences relating to source of
diagnostic material (Minna, 1982). Squamous cell carcinoma is the
most frequently diagnosed histologic type, from both surgical   resection and from biopsy or cytology material. Generally, however, a-
denocarcinoma is diagnosed mainly from surgical resection in relation
to the more frequent peripheric localization (Berg, 1982; Jett, 1983)
while espholiative-type tumours (squamous cell) and those which are
often more central, such as squamous cell and SCCL, are diagnosed

more frequently from citology material or bronchial biopsy (Berg,
1982; Geddes, 1984). SCCL appears more often on autopsy reports since
presumably patients die rapidly without having a prior diagnosis.
d- Distribution by age group of the different histologic types is,
on the other hand, homogenous with the exception of adenocarcinoma
of which there is an earlier incidence in younger women (Greenberg,
1984).

The factors outlined above emphasize the difficulties in interpretat
ing data, particularly from hospital series with changes in criteria
of access to services, case selection etc. Despite this, an extensive
comparison of data from many parts of the world allows us to identify
several general features.

Table 6 and 7 show distribution in both sexes of SCCL as shown in po
pulation-based Cancer Registries in various parts of the world in recent years.
The frequency of SCCL in Italy is around 10%, from 10.1 in Latina to
12.1% in Florence, for both sexes. The values are therefore low, like
those of some areas in Asia and Israel, compared with those registered
in other zones (USA, Canada, Hungary and Poland).

TABLE 6   Percentage of Small Cell Cancer of the Lung
(SCCL) by Sex in some Population based Studies   in
Europe

Area and Years of Observation	N. cases *	Confirm. Istol. %	M/F	SCCL% ** Males	Females
County Vas (H) 1973-82	1201	68.5	7.0	20.4	18.9
Saarland (FRG) 1974-83	5738	58.6	8.0	22.3	32.5
Parma (I) 1977-83	1580	62.2	-	11.5*	
Vaud (CH) 1977-84	2838	-	6.5	17.1	16.7
Bas-Rhinois (F) 1978-81	1284	91.0	-	13.2*	
Varese (I) 1978-81	1672	38.2	9.1	10.7	16.2
Krakow N.Sacz (PL) 1978-83	2597	50.6	4.5	18.5	24.4
Scotland (UK) 1980-84	23116	-	2.5	11.2	15.5
Latina (I) 1982-85	474	52.1	9.3	10.2	9.5
Florence (I) 1984	647	62.6	6.4	12.0	13.0
Trent (UK) 1984-85	6874	53.3	-	17.7*	

* males and females
**only cases with histologic confirmation

TABLE 7   Percentage of Small Cell Cancer of the Lung (SCCL) by Sex in some Population-Based Studies in the World (Excluded Europe).

Area and Years of Observation	No Cases *	Confirm. Istolog.%	M/F	SCCL % ** Males	Females
Israel 1961-72	5330	68.0	3.0	11.5	9.1
Osaka 1967-78	13037	37.1	3.4**	10.3	8.0
Singapore 1968-72	7786	60.2	2.8	7.1*	
Alberta (Canada) 1972-81	5301	93.5	-	18.1*	
N.Hampsh.-Vermont 1973-76 (USA)	1906	82.9	3.9	19.8	27.6
USA 1973-77	45836	86.8	2.8	14.0	16.6
Hong Kong 1977-80	3192	55.8	2.3	22.6	20.9
USA 1977-81	6063**	-	2.1**	17.3	19.3
South Australia 1977-85	4504	-	4.3	15.9	17.6
Ontario (Canada) 1979-83	21140	73.1	-	19.2*	
New South Wales 1980-82 (Australia)	6117	-	3.9	15.5	21.8
Canada *** 1981	11576	75.5	3.1	14.0	15.5
New Zealand 1981-82	2589	69.3	2.9	14.4	21.8
New Brunswick 1983-84 (Canada)	777	-	-	14.0*	
Shangai (China)**** feb.1984-feb.1985	1221	-	1.2	9.3	6.3
Manibota (Canada) 1984-85	1310	-	-	16.6*	

* males and females
** only cases with histologic confirmation
*** excluded data of Manibota Cancer Registry
**** only age-class 35-64.

Table 8 shows SCCL percentage in males in several hospital-based studies. This percentages are higher than those in population-based studies and this is probably due to the different selection of cases.

TABLE 8 Percentage of Small Cell Cancer of the Lung
(SCCL) in Males in Some Hospital-based   Studies.

....

Author, Year of Publication	Year of Observat.	No Cases	SCCL %
Yesner, 1973 *	1953-59	449	21.8
Cox, 1979	1958-77	1017	22.2
Vincent, 1977	1962-75	1404	18.2
Kung, 1984 **	1973-82	714	21.3
Shimizu, 1986	1977-82	661	15.7
Liberati, 1983 *	1978-79	1692	18.5
Delendi, unpubl.**	1979-80	346	35.8
Celikoglu, 1986	1979-83	324	29.6
Buiatti, 1985	1981-83	340	12.1

....

* males and females
**cases from Pathology Department.

TRENDS BY HISTOLOGIC TYPE

The interpretation of incidence trends involves problems due to chan
ges, through time, in the registration rules and in particular, in
the development of diagnostic methods. Other difficulties relate to
studies on trends by particular histologic types; variability through
time can, in fact, depend on a series of factors, namely:
1. Distribution by age-group particularly important in adenocarcinoma
in women.
2. Percentage of histologic confirmation, which varies from country
to country and never reaches 100%. The SCCL percentages reported in
Tables 6 and 7 are calculated on the basis only of a series with hist
ologic confirmation and not on the total number of cases.
3. Differences attribuitable to pathologists who have defined   the
histologic types: variability having been documented in several studies (Hanai, 1987; Yesner, 1973).
4. Introduction of new laboratory diagnostic techniques(Wu, 1986)
5. The use of different classification systems: this has to be carefully considered, expecially in the evaluation of temporal trends
which take into account data registered before 1968, year in which
the MOTNAC system was introduced. Before that, generally "small cell
carcinoma" was classified together with "large cell carcinoma" and
"oat cell carcinoma" was classified together with "anaplastic carcinoma" (Berg, 1982; Wu, 1986).
Even considering these difficulties, several authors have studied sin
gle series to check for changes in the frequency of histologic types
over the years. In particular:
Vincent (1977) examined a series of 1682 patients relating to the pe
riod 1962-75. While the SCCL trend showed to be consistently stable,
there was an increase in adenocarcinoma and a decrease in squamous
cell carcinoma.
Also Hanai and colleagues   (1982), examining the series registered

at the Osaka Cancer Registry between 1967-78 showed an increase in
adenocarcinoma and a decrease in squamous cell carcinoma. SCCL, although based on small numbers, was higher both in males and females
in recent years (5.0% in 1967-72 and 11.8% in 1973-78 for males; 5.1%
in 1967-72 and 8.7% in 1973-78 for females).
Geddes and others (1984), describing a series of 1986 cases relating
to the period 1971-81, demonstrated a significant increase in the per
centage of squamous cell carcinomas and a decrease in adenocarcinomas
both in males and females. There was also a decrease, although not
significant, in SCCL.
In 1986 Dodds and others published data relating to the cases register
ed between 1974 and 1981 by the Cancer Surveillance System of the
Fred Hutchinson Cancer Research Centre, one of the ten population bas
ed Cancer Registries which operate under the NCI SEER Program. As
shown in Table 9, annual rates in both sexes show only a slight increase.

TABLE 9   Annual Incidence Rates of SCCL x 100,000
inh. (Standard: 1970 U.S. Population - Dodds, 1986)

Year	Rate	
	Males	Females
1974	9.9.	3.5
1975	8.6	3.5
1976	10.5	4.4
1977	12.1	4.4
1978	13.8	6.7
1979	11.3	5.6
1980	11.1	4.7
1981	12.3	5.6

Berg and co-workers (1982) examined several USA series relating to
the period 1949-77, a period in which there was an increase in lung
cancer incidence in both sexes. There was a change in sex ratio for
lung cancer on the whole and by single histologic type. The change
was greater for SCCL which showed a higher increase for females. This
increase was believed not to be influenced by variations in diagnost
ic tecniques and classification criteria as these would have had a
similar effect on both sexes.
In Table 10 and 11 we have reported relative frequencies in various
histologic types in series relating to different time period. This
overall view shows that, although SCCL frequency appears in many cases
to be higher in more recent years, because the relatively small number of cases, the figures are not consistent.

RISK FACTORS RELATED TO SCCL

Cigarette smoking is the major risk factor correlated to lung cancer,
this correlation having by now been sufficiently proven in literature.

TABLE 10   Relative   Frequencies of the Major   Lung Cancer Histologic Types in Males in Some   Selected Population-Based Studies

Area	Time Period	No Cases	Histologic Types %			
			Squam.	SCCL	Adenoc.	Others
Osaka	1967-72	614	54.7	5.0	29.8	10.5
(Japan)	1973-78	2273	44.7	11.8	35.3	8.2
USA	1974-77	2810	35.6	15.4	22.3	26.7
	1978-81	3318	33.5	17.4	27.4	21.7
Vaud (CH)	1977-80	1204	46.0	16.3	9.7	28.0
	1981-84	1257	42.2	18.0	15.9	23.9
Saarland	1974-78	2593	35.1	12.0	3.7	49.2
(FRG)	1979-83	2511	33.1	14.6	5.8	46.5
County Vas	1973-77	498	54.9	27.7	5.5	11.9
(H)	1978-82	553	50.8	13.4	11.2	24.6

TABLE 11   Relative Frequencies of the   Major Lung Cancer Histologic Types in Females in Some Selected Population-Based Studies

Area	Time Period	No Cases	Histologic Types %			
			Squam.	SCCL	Adenoc.	Others
Osaka	1967-72	156	29.8	5.1	56.4	8.7
(Japan)	1973-78	686	23.0	8.7	59.8	8.5
USA	1974-77	1146	19.5	16.7	35.8	28.0
	1978-81	1623	19.0	20.0	38.1	22.9
Vaud (CH)	1977-80	162	14.8	11.7	35.2	38.3
	1981-84	215	15.3	20.5	32.6	31.6
Saarland	1974-78	284	19.7	16.2	10.2	53.9
	1979-83	350	12.9	18.6	15.1	53.4

Towards the mid 1950's, Kreyberg proposed a classification of the various histologic types of lung cancer into two etiological groups. The first group, correlated to exposure to inhalants such as tobacco smoke, constitutes squamous cell carcinoma, SCCL and large cell carcinoma. The second group constitutes the other histologic types, including adenocarcinoma, not correlated to exposure to tobacco smoke. This theory, supported by Doll(1957), is consistent with results from some studies (Archer, 1974; Koo, 1985 - only in males; Yesner, 1973), but not from others (Morton, 1982; Stayner, 1983; Weiss, 1972). With regard to SCCL, the correlation with tobacco smoke has been found to be stronger compared to the other histologic types and, in males, to be related to the dose inhaled (Stayner, 1983; Weiss, 1972, Yesner, 1973).

Today it is generally believed that all histologic types have smoking in common as a risk factor, although it may be at different levels.

To interpret trends by histologic type and to forecast a possible trend in lung cancer (and SCCL) in future decades, it is necessary to know the diffusion of smoking in the population and the composition of cigarettes on the market.

There is a progressive increase in cigarette sales in Italy from 1968 to 1983. This is contrary to other European countries in which there has been a recent decrease (U.K., USA, West Germany, Denmark) (IARC, 1986).

With regard to residual tar content, cigarettes sold in Italy are "heavy" cigarettes with a quantity of tar among the highest in Europe (IARC, 1986).

With regard to other environmental carcinogens, Table 12 shows SCCL frequency distribution in several occupational categories.

This percentage varies from 10.6% in blue collar workers (Stayner, 1983) to 61.7% in uranium miners (Archer, 1974), reaching a figure of 12 cases of SCCL out of 13 lung cancer exposed to chloromethyl methyl ether (Figueroa, 1973).

TABLE 12   Percentage of   Small   Cell   Lung Cancer
(SCCL) in Selected Occupational   Studies

Author, Year of public.	Occupational Categories	No Cases	SCCL %
Archer, 1974	uranium miners	107	61.7
Newman, 1976	copper smelters	25	28.0
	copper miners	54	20.4
Whitwell, 1974	workers affected from asbestosis	97	26.8
Stayner, 1983	blue collars	292	10.6
	white collars	128	10.9
Vallyathan, 1985 (modified)	coal miners	171	26.0

SURVIVAL

It is   known that survival from lung cancer, an area which has seen very few changes in recent years, depends on a series of factors, including age and stage of illness (Adelstein, 1981; Horm, 1984; Temeck, 1984). Nevertheless, one of the fundamental contributing factors is the histologic type. Tables 13 and 14 show survival rates based respectively on a series of clinic trials (Jackson, 1986) and on a population study (Mould, 1982). The data are extremely diversified. The less positive results of Table 13 (Trial II, with a survival to two years of 13.7%)exceeds the one year survival shown in the population

study (survival to one year of 13.5%). On the one hand, this demonstrates the difficulty of extrapolating trials results to the whole
population, as groups of selected patients are still involved. On the
other hand, it would seem to point out that one aim, in public health
terms, must be transfer any positive results which have been achieved
in centres of special capacity, to the population as a whole.

TABLE 13 Two-Year   Survival in Different   Trials
(Jackson, 1986).

| Trial | No. of Patients | | | | | | 2-yr Survival (Estimated % ±SE) |
| | Overall | | Limited Disease | | Extensive Disease | | |
	Tot.	CR*	Tot.	CR*	Tot.	CR*	
I	11	7	7	4	4	3	20.4±5.5
II	14	14	7	7	7	7	13.7±3.4
III	19	17	16	14	3	3	17.4±3.2
CAV	9	7	9	7	0	0	13.9±4.0
VCAV	10	10	7	7	3	3	21.4±4.8
IV	3	3	3	3	0	0	31.5±7.9

* Patients with Complete Response (CR) to the therapy.

TABLE 14   Crude and Relative Percentage   Survival
Rates of Histologically Proven Treated Lung Cancer,
by Sex and Histological Group ($\pm$ s.e. is given in
brackets for each crude survival rate) (Mould, 1982)

Sex	Histology	No Cases	1-year Survival Crude	Rates (%) Relative
Male	Squam. cell ca.	1037	39.1 (±1.5)	41.2
"	Adenocarcinoma	164	36.0 (±3.8)	37.3
"	Oat cell ca.*	238	13.5 (±2.2)	14.0
Female	Squam. cell ca.	311	34.6 (±2.7)	35.4
"	Adenocarcinoma	90	28.9 (±4.8)	29.5
"	Oat cell ca. *	196	14.0 (±2.5)	14.3

* Other subtypes of SCCL are excluded

CONCLUSIONS

On the basis of this report, we can present some hypothesis in respon
se to the question about SCCL incidence and mortality increase:
a- The survey of data from various series and from Cancer Registries
does not provide an univocal answer as regards SCCL increase. Never-

theless, in many series, the SCCL percentage in recent periods has been higher than it was previously.

b- In several countries, and particularly in Italy, there is an increase in lung cancer incidence and mortality which presumably will continue in the future. The number of SCCL is therefore bound to increase.

c- The survival of patients affected by SCCL is lower than that of subjects with other types of lung cancer. Therapeutic improvements in few situations cannot easily be applied to the total population. Thus an increase in SCCL incidence, greater than that for other histologic types, is bound to result in a significant further increase in lung cancer mortality.

ACKNOWLEDGEMENT

The authors would like to express their gratitude to the Cancer Regis tries of Alberta (Canada), Bas-Rhinois (F), County Vas (H), Israel, Krakow and Nowy Sacz (PL), Latina (I), Manibota (Canada), New Brunsw ick (Canada), New Foundland(Canada), New South Wales (Australia), New Zealand, Nova Scotia (Canada), Ontario (Canada), Osaka (Japan), Parma (I), Prince Edward Island (Canada), Quebec (Canada), Ragusa (I), Saar land (FRG), Saskatchewan (Canada), Scotland (UK), Seattle (USA), Shan gai (China), Singapore ,   South Australia, Trent (UK), Trieste (I), Varese (I), Vaud (CH) and the National Cancer Incidence System of Canada. Portion of the data are obtained for this paper from these sources.

REFERENCES

Adelstein, A.M., and others(1981).Cancer Statistics. Incidence. Survi val and Mortality in England and Wales. Hobbbs, London.

Archer, V.E., G. Saccomanno, and J.H. Jones (1974). Frequency of different histologic types of bronchogenic carcinoma as related to ra diation exposure. Cancer, 34, 2056-2060.

Berg, J.W., C. Percy, and J.W Horm (1982). Recent changes in the Pat tern of occurrence of Oat (ll Carcinoma of the Lung. In K.Magnus (Ed.), Trends in Cancer Incidence, Hemisphere, USA, 215-221.

Buiatti E., and others (1985). A case-control study of lung cancer in Florence, Italy. I Occupational risk factors. J. Epid.Com. H.,39, 244-250.

Cancer Statistics (1985). Ca-A Cancer J. Clin. vol., 35, 1, New York.

Capocaccia, R., and others (1984). La mortalità in Italia nel periodo 1970-79. ISTISAN, Roma.

Capocaccia, R., and others (1985). La mortalità in Italia nell'anno 1980. ISTISAN, Roma

Capocaccia, R., and others (1986). La mortalità in Italia nell'anno 1981. ISTISAN, Roma

Celikoglu, S.I., and others (1986). Frequency of distribution according to histological types of lung cancer in the tracheobronchial tree. Respiration, 49, 152-156.

Cox, J.D., R.A. Yesner (1979). Adenocarcinoma of the lung: recent resul ts from the Veterans Administration Lung Group. Am.Rev.Respir.Dis.,

120, 1025-1029

Dodds, L., S. Davis, and L. Polissar (1986). A population-based study of lung cancer incidence trends by histologic type, 1974-81.J.N.C.I., 76(1), 21-28.

Doll, R., B. Hill, L. Kreyberg (1957). The significance of cell type in relation to the etiology of lung cancer. Br.J. Cancer, 11, 43-48

Doll, R. (1982). Trends in mortality from lung cancer in women. in K. Magnus (Ed.) Trends in Cancer Incidence, Hemisphere, USA, 223-230.

Figueroa, W.G., R. Raszkòwski, and W. Weiss (1973). Lung cancer in clhoromethyl methyl ether workers. New Engl.J.Med., 288, 1096-1097.

Geddes, M., and others (1984). Cell type distribution in histologic specimens of primary lung cancer. Tumori, 70, 255-260

Greenberg, E.R., and others (1984). Incidence of lung cancer by cell type: a population-based study in New Hampshire and Vermont.J.N.C.I; 72(3), 599-603.

Hanai, A., and others (1982). Trends of lung cancer incidence and their histological distribution in Osaka. Communication, 13th International Cancer Congress, Seattle.

Hanai, A., and others (1987). Concordance of histological classification of lung cancer with special reference to adenocarcinoma in Osaka, Japan, and the North-West Region of England. Int.J.Cancer,39, 6-9.

Horm, J.W., and others (1984). Cancer incidence and Mortality in the U.S. SEER, 1973-81. NIH Publ., Bethesda.

Horm, J.W., and L.G. Kessler (1986). Falling rates of lung cancer in men in the United States. Lancet (The), 8478(1), 425-426.

IARC Monograph (1986). Evalutation of the Carcinogenic Risk of Chemicals to Humans. Tobacco Smoking, IARC, Vol. 38, Lyon.

Jackson, D.V.Jr., and L.D. Case, (1986). Small cell lung cancer: a 10 years perspective. Seminars in Oncology. 13(3), 63-74.

Jett, J.R., D.A. Cortese, and R.S. Fontana, (1983). Lung cancer: current concepts and prospects. Cancer J.Clin., 33(2), 74-85.

Klaassen, D.J., and others (1986). Is lung cancer a sexist disease? Communication, 14th International Cancer Congress, Budapest.

Koo, L.C, J.H-C.Ho, and N. Lee, (1985). An analysis of some risk factors for lung cancer in Hong Kong. Int.J.Cancer, 35, 149-155.

Kung, I.T.M., K.F.So, and T.H.Lam (1984). Lung cancer in Hong Kong Chinese: Mortality and histological types, 1973-1982. Br.J.Cancer, 50, 381-388.

Kvale, G. (1982). Incidence trends in the Nordic Countries. In K. Magnus (Ed.) Trends in Cancer Incidence. Hemisphere, USA 185-197.

Liberati, A., and others (1983). Lung cancer care in general hospitals. Tumori, 69, 567-573.

Minna, J.D., G.A. Higgins, and E.J.Glatstein (1982). Cancer of the lung. In V.T. De Vita (Ed.) Cancer Principles and Practice of Oncology. Lippincott Company, Philadelphia.

Morton, W.E., and E.L. Treyve (1982). Histologic differences in occupational risks of lung cancer incidence. Am.J.Ind.Med.,3,441-457.

Mould, R.F., and R.J.Williams (1982). Survival of histologically proven carcinoma of the lung registered in the North West Thames Region 1975-79. Br.J.Cancer, 46, 999-1003.

Newman, J.A., and others (1976). Histologic type of bronchogenic car

cinoma among members of copper-minig and smelting communities. In
  Academy of Science (Ed.). <u>Occupational Carcinogens</u>, New York
Shimizu, H., and others (1986). Risk of lung cancer by histologic
  type among smokers in Miyagi Prefecture. <u>Jpn. J.Cl.Oncol.</u>, <u>16(2)</u>,
  117-121.
Stayner, L.T., and D.H.Wegman (1983). Smoking, occupation and histo-
  pathology of lung cancer: a case-control study with the use of the
  Third National Cancer Survey. <u>J.N.C.I.</u>, <u>70(3)</u>, 421-426.
Temeck, B.K., B.J.Flehinger, and N. Martini (1984). A retrospective
  Analysis of 10-year survivors from carcinoma of the lung. <u>Cancer</u>,53,
  1405-1408.
Vallyathan, V., and others (1985). Lung carcinoma by histologic type
  in coal miners. <u>Arch.Pathol.Lab.Med.</u>, <u>109</u>, 419-423.
Vincent, R.G., and others (1977). The changing histopathology of lung
  cancer. A review of 1682 cases. <u>Cancer, 39,</u> 1647-1655.
Weiss, W., and others (1972). Risk of lung cancer according to histologic type and cigarette dosage. <u>J.A.M.A.</u>,<u>222(7)</u>, 799-801.
Whitwell, F., M.L.Newhouse, and D.R.Bcnnet (1974). A study of the
  histological cell types of lung cancer in workers suffering from
  asbestosis in the United Kingdom. <u>Br.J.Ind.Med.</u>, <u>31,</u> 298-303.
Wu, A.H., and others (1986). Secular trends in histologic types of
  lung cancer. <u>J.N.C.I.</u>, <u>77(1),</u> 53-56.
Yesner, R., N.A. Gelfman, and A.R. Fenstein (1973). A reappraisal of
  histopathology in lung cancer and correlation of cell types with
  antecedent cigarette smoking. <u>Am.Review Resp.Dis.</u>, <u>107</u>, 790-797.
Young J.L., and others (1981). Cancer Incidence and mortality in the
  U.S., 1973-77. Natl. Cancer Inst. Monogr., <u>57</u>, 1-1082.

The Pathology of Small Cell Lung Cancer (SCLC): Diagnostic and Prognostic Significance of New Technical Approaches

V. Tison*, G. Rosti[†] G. Caruso*,
O. Fiscelli* E. Govoni[‡] F. Morigi* and
M. Marangolo[†]

*Servizio di Anatomia Patologica, Osp. "Maurizio
Bufalini", USL 39 Cesena;
[†]Oncologia Medica, Osp. "S. Maria delle Croci" USL
35, Ravenna;
[‡]Istituto di Microscopia Elettronica Clinica, Università
di Bologna, Policlcinico S. Orsola, Italy

ABSTRACT

Histologically the SCLC is divided in three subtypes:intermediate variant; small and large cell variant; oat-cell variant. The last is only the result of ischemic-necrotic alterations born in the contest of the intermediate one. The SCLC is a neuroendocrine neoplasia strictly correlated with the carcinoid and the atypical carcinoid with which have to be separated from the morphological and clinical point of view.

The Authors are convinced that few types of cells are able in the lung to give place to SCLC and have observed that some small neoplastic cell can produce at the same time dense-core granules,keratin, and lamellar citosomes.

KEYWORDS

SCLC, carcinoid, atypical carcinoid, ultrastructure, histogenesis, intermediate, oat-cell, neuroendocrine, lung.

Four principal histological types of lung carcinoma are at present distinguished by WHO: epidermoid carcinoma; adenocarcinoma; large cell carcinoma; small cell carcinoma (SCLC). While the last two look undifferentiaded under the optical microscope, the ultrastructure has demonstrated that the truly undifferentiated cases are very rare(NOMORI and co-workers,1986).On one side the SCLC has the aspect of an APUD cell neoplasia, while on the other side the large cell carcinoma has many features in common with other types of lung malignancies.

From the clinical and practical point of view the lung carcinomas may be divided in two main categories: the small cell carcinoma(SCLC) and the non-small cell carcinoma(N-SCLC). The SCLC is infact a clearly distinct, and anatomical entity,representing 25% of all human lung

maligniancies(Gazdar,1986). The epithelial nature of the SCLC was recognized in 1926 by Barnard and in 66% of the cases it arises from
the main bronchi as a whitish tissue, slightly protruding from the
mucosal surface and invading, in an iceberg fashion, the surrounding
structures particularly the vessels, precociously involved.

The neuroendocrine nature of the SCLC is well known since 1966,
strictly akin to that of the carcinoids, of which the SCLC represen-
tes the more aggressive and the less differentiated counterpert. From
this derives the proposal to use the common term of neuroendocrine
tumor for all these tumors, specifyng case by case the degree of differentiation: carcinoid, atypical carcinoid and SCLC or KCC-I, KCC-II,
KCC-III(respectively)(Paladugu and co-workers,1985).

Histologically the SCLC is divided in three subtypes(Carter and
Yesner,1985):
A) the intermediate variant;
B) the small and large cell carcinoma;
C) the oat cell carcinoma.

Before describing the histological features of the SCLC it is necessary to recall how frequent classification mistakes are due to the
crush artifacts caused by the bioptic sampling on a necrotic and fra-
gile neoplastic tissue. Perhaps 20% of the SCLC diagnosis is incorrect
(Yesner,1986) being a different subtype,or a limphoma or, sometimes,
a phlogistic infiltration. Moreover the surgical or autoptical specimens have shown that in a large percentage the SCLC is associated
with different types of carcinoma (see below), particularly epidermoid, glandular and true carcinoid (Mattheus and Gazdar,1982;Brereton
and co-workers,1978;Yesner,1985;Burdon,Sinclair and Henderson,1979).
This is not surprising due to the in vitro ability of the SCLC to
differentiate all the other types of lung carcinomas (but not the re-
verse), while the same epidermoid carcinoma in the long dating cultures give rise to glandular structures (Gazdar,1986;Kameya,Kodama and
Shimosata,1982).

Lastly it is mandatory to underline that the oat cell variant is
now considered only the result of ischemic and necrotic modifications
arising in the common intermediate variant(Gazdar,1986). This is in
accord with the clinical-biological behaviour of these two subtypes,
completely similar(Hansen and co-workers,1978).Therefore a short mention will be given of the oat cell variant, and even of the combined
one (SCLC plus adenocarcinoma and squamous carcinomas) still considered separated by some pathologistis.

SCLC -Intermediate variant

This is the most common subtype of SCLC, about 70-90%. The cells
form ribbons, festoons or solid areas, often with interponing fields
of necrosis and pseudorosette structures. The cells are poligonal or
spindle shaped from two to four times the size of a limphocyte (Carter and Yesner,1985)(fig.1). While the cytoplasm shows no differentiation, the nuclei are slightly irregular, round or spindle, with a
chromatin pattern evenly distributed. The nucleoli are not as frequent and large, or at least prominent,as in the atypical carcinoid,
a form with the differential diagnosis could be very difficult. Even
the chromatin pattern in the latter is more irregular than in SCLC
(fig.2). To be noted however that the atypical carcinoid is most of-

ten a peripheral lesion.

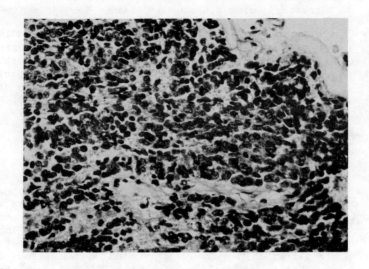

Fig. 1: SCLC Intermediate variant. Solid area with
necrosis and pseudorosettes.Hemat.Eos.240x

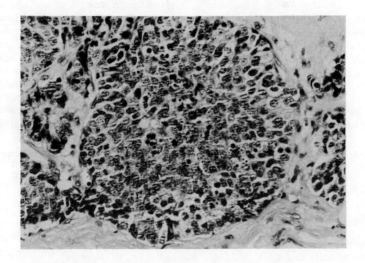

Fig. 2: Atypical carcinoid.The nuclei have irregular
chromatin and evident nucleoli.Hemat.Eos.400x

The argyrophilia is always negative, although the ultrastructure of most of these cells demonstrates dense core granules, however less numerous, smaller and more irregular in size than in either the typical or atypical carcinoid(Carter and Yesner,1985)(fig.3).

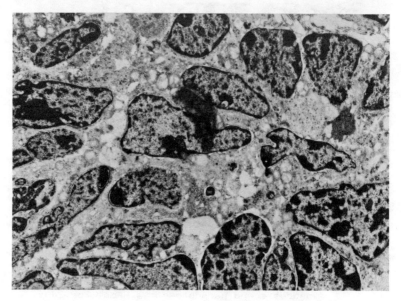

Fig. 3: SCLC. The regular dense core granules are
not so numerous as in carcinoid.3800x

In the cytological preparations the SCLC is tipycal: bands or clusters of small cells with predominanting round or oval nuclei having an homogeneous or finely granular chromatin, while the nucleoli are small or not visible. The cells on a necrotic ground mould one on the other forming piles or clusters in which they often form 45°' angles.

SCLC-Small/large cell variant.

This type makes about 20% of SCLC, and is formed by the combination of small cells, like that of the intermediate variant, with large cells having abundant cytoplasm and prominent vescicular nuclei with big nucleoli(Carter and Yesner,1985)(fig.4).

Radice and co-workers,1982, identified this subtype because in an homogeneous group of patients treated in the same way it was more often found in an advanced stage at the time of the first diagnosis and subsequently was less respondent to therapy.

The metastates are often formed only by the small cell counterpart(Carter and Yesner,1985) and the endocrine differentiation is less frequent than in the other variants(Gazdar,1984). In vitro cultures of pure SCLC dating back since two years very ofeten give rise to a large component seemingly representing the result of a long standing growth(Gazdar and co-workers,1981).

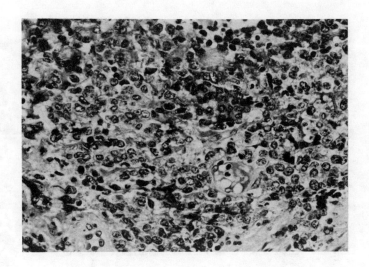

Fig. 4: SCLC small/large variant. A combination of
        small cell, of intermediate variant with
        larger elements with abundant cytoplasm,ve-
        scicular nuclei and evident nucleoli.Hemat.
        Eos.400x

The discovery of Little and co-workers,1983, that an amplified
c-myc oncogene is espressed by this variant leads to think that it
represents a distinct biological entity and not a casual combination
of two different subtypes.

SCLC combined with squamous or adenocarcinoma.
    In many series(Abeloff and co-workers,1979;Matthews,1979;Yesner,
Auerbach and Gerste,1979) the association between SCLC and different
neoplastic histotypes is underlined, with a percentage ranging from
15% to 20% or even 33%(Gazdar and co-workers,1984). This is an important point due to the fact that this variant, like the small/large
cell carcinoma combination does not show the same responsiveness to
chemotherapy and radiotherapy as the "pure SCLC"(Carter and Yesner,1985).

Oat cell variant.
    Sometimes this term is used as a synonymous of SCLC, but more
properly is referred to the lymphocyte-like variant, which is 1-1/2
to two times the diameter of a lymphocyte(Carter and Yesner,1985).Ne-
crosis and regressive changes are the stigmata of this subtype, being
the oat cell pratically formed only by"naked" and homogeneous nuclei,
sometimes with a small rim of cytoplasm,moulding one on the other(fig.5).
    This variant, mainly recognized on bioptic material deeply modi-

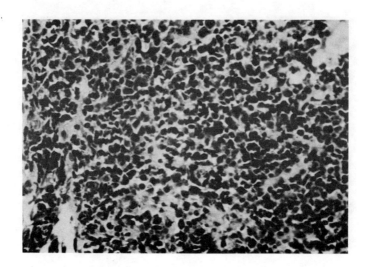

Fig. 5: SCLC, oat cell variant. Uniform field of small
homogeneous and necrotic cell.Hemat.Eos.400x

fied by crush artifacts, is now better considered only the product
of necrotic ischemic modifications born in the usual and much more
frequent intermediate subtype. Thereafter it looks in someway artifi-
cious any attempt of subtle analysis of the chromatin pattern which
is described as smooth, evenly distribuited with small and indistinct
nucleoli, rarely seen.

DIFFERENTIAL DIAGNOSIS BETWEEN SCLC, CARCINOID AND ATYPICAL
CARCINOID.

Carcinoid: is identified by argirophilia, ultrasrtuctural evidence of dense-core granules and good prognosis(Carter and Yesner,
1985). More often arising from the proximal bronchial tree the carcinoid can even be peripheral, sometimes having an extrapulmonary
expansion. It grows as a polypoid smooth,sessile, endobronchial mass.
The cells are polygonal or spindle, with an evident, granular eosinophilic cytoplasm, while the nuclei are round or oval having promi-
nenti or at least evident nucleoli on a granular chromatinic ground.
Ribbons, festoons and frequently pseudorosettes are the histoarchi-
tectural pattern of carcinoids being not rare the mucin production
and the papillary projection (fig.6).
    The peripheral small carcinoids are called "tumorlets", frequen-
tly multiple and in scar borning(Whitwell,1955).
    Neurofilaments and neuron-specific enolase(Lehto and co-workers,
1984; Gould and co-workers, 1983) are constantly present while a vast

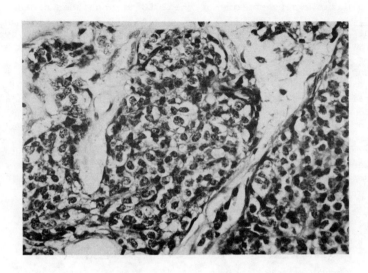

Fig. 6: Carcinoid. Typical field of cells with abundant, granular, eosinophilic cytoplasm and
a round nucleus. Hemat.Eos.400x

range of hormones is produced, like ACTH, calcitonin, bombesin, insulin, GRP and so on (Yang and co-workers, 1983; Kamai and co-workers, 1983).

Atypical carcinoid: It is more often a peripheral neoplasm gi-
ving rise to metastasis in 60% of cases, with a prognosis intermediate between that of carcinoid and that of SCLC, while the mortality rate is 35% (Carter and Yesner, 1985). The histoarchitecture
is the same of carcinoid, but with necrosis, numerous mitotic figures and more atypical nuclei. The biological properties are that of
carcinoids, producing calcitonin, bombesin, and NSE. Neurofilaments
are often visible while the dense-core granules are less numerous
and more varied in size than in typical carcinoid, but not so rare
as in SCLC.
The nuclei are similar to that of an adenocarcinoma, larger,
more irregular than in carcinoid, with prominent nucleoli. However,
the chromatin pattern is not so homogeneous, evenly distributed as
in SCLC.
In summary the atypical carcinoid is a carcinoma distinguished
from carcinoid by the necrosis and from SCLC by the chromatin pattern (Paladugu and co-workers, 1985).

SCLC - Histogenesis
Saying first of all that only one stem-cell is thought to be
at beginning of all the types of lung carcinomas(Gazdar,1986),we

have to admit that this seems to us more a philosophical concept,
than a concret one: what is indeed the stem cell? Having examined
all the putative progenitors of the SCLC we concluded prefering a
multidirectional differentiation histogenesis (tumors with an endocrine phenotype may arise from non-endocrine cell - i.e. hypothe-
tical stem cell, indifferent/intermediate cell derived from basal
cell or small mucous granule cell - which have been driven by micro-
environmental pathologic factors toward expressing an endocrine cell
phenotype).

It is in fact our opinion that in many neoplastic and non neoplastic condition cells from different structures can give rise to
neuroendocrine elements. For instance we have found a "third" type
ofpneumocyte emerging in the alveoli of strong smokers, producing
at the same time dense core granules, lamellar cytosomes and cytokeratins.

Completely similar cell, we have discovered in some SCLC(fig.7).

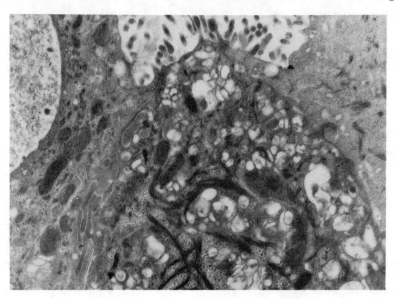

Fig. 7: SCLC. A neoplastic cell with dense core gra-
        nules, cytokeratin filaments and lamellar
        cytosomes. 18.000x

In conclusion there is today a general agreement in considering
the SCLC the most aggressive, undifferentiated side of a neoplastic
process that starting from native cells gives rise,according to the
degree of differentiation, to carcinoid, atypical carcinoid and SCLC
(Gazdar,1986; Paladugu and co-workers,1985).

In fact, even if non argyrophilic the SCLC very often produces
not only bombesin, L-Dopa decarbossilase and chromogranin(Gazdar,
1986), but also all the range of hormonesjust mentioned as typical
of carcinoids (ACTH, calcitonin, serotonin, somatostatin, AVP, etc.)

(Bondy and Gilby,1982;Kasurinen and Syrjanen,1986). Often the secretion is multihormonal (Hattori and co-workers), while it is not rare
a clear cut positivity for the leucoenkephalin, the NSE(Wick and co-
workers,1983; Gould and co workres,1983) and the sera monoclonal MOV
15 and K1 67.

To be recalled that SCLC is associated with a specific deletion
of the 14-23 region of the short arm of chromosom 3(Whang-Peng and
co-workers,1982), which corresponds tothe aminociclasi gene, and with
varying and different types of oncogene amplifications (c-myc,L-myc,
N-myc)(Gazdar,1986;Little and co-workers,1983). These markers seem
to be more strictly related with the biological activities of these
tumors than is the neuroendocrine differentiation(Carter and Yesner).
For instance the prognosis looks poore when c-myc oncogene is
evident (Gazdar,1986).

It was reported that DNA-content of SCLC is aneuploid(Bum and
co-workers,1983) in 83% of cases, and that SCLC lines have a markedly
deficient or absent expression of HLA-A, B and C framework proteins
and B-2 microglobulins(Doyle and Cuttitta,1983).
Finally, SCLC keratin content is variable, mainly consisting of
small molecular weight forms, while the vimentin is lacking(Carney
and Gazdar,1986).

ACKNOWLEDGEMENT

The lecture was partly based on the histological material kin-
dly provided by the collegues: M. De Maurizi (Imola Hosp.);E.Magni
(Ravenna Hosp.);R. Ferracini (Bellaria Hosp., Bologna); M.Mariuzzi
(Ancona University); A.Saragoni (Forlì Hosp.); G.Scilabra (Lugo
Hosp.).
Theauthors are particularly indebeted to the technician Mister
Giovanni Benedettini for the accurate histological preparations.

REFERENCES

Abeloff,M.D., J.C.Eggleston, G.Mendelsohn and co-workers(1979).Chan-
ges in morphologic and biochemical characteristics of small cell
carcinoma of the lung. Am.J.Med.,66, 757-764.
Barnad,W.G.(1926). The nature of the "oat-cell sarcoma" of the mediastinum. J.Pathol.Bact.,29,241-244.
Bondy,P.K. and E.D.Gilby(1982). Peptide hormone immunoreactivity and
prognosis in small cell carcinoma of the lung.Respiration,49,61-67.
Brereton,H.D.,M.J.Matthews,J.Costa and co-workers(1978). Mixed anaplastic small cell and squamous-cell carcinoma of the lung.Am.In-
tern.Med.,8, 805-806.
Burdon J.G.W., R.A.Sinclair and M.M.Henderson(1979). Small cell carcinoma of the lung. Prognosis in relation to histological subtype.
Chest.,76,302-304.
Bum,P.A., D.H.Carney,A.F.Gazdar and co-workers(1983). Diagnostic and
biological implications of flow cytometric DNA content analysis in
lung cancer. Cancer Res.,43,5032-5038.
Carney,D.N. and A.F.Gadzar(1986).Unpublished data. In A.F.Gazdar,Is-

26   V. Tison *et al.*

tocitopatologia,8,151-158.

Carter,D.C. and R.Yesner.(1985). Carcinomas of the lung with neuroendocrine differentiation. Seminars in Diagnostic Pathology,2,235-
254.

Doyle,A.,A.F.Cuttitta(1983). Small cell lung cancer lines differ
markedly in the exspression of HLA-framework and B-2 microglobu
lin antigens(abstracts). Proc.Am.Soc.Clin.Oncol.,2,12-

Gazdar,A.F.,D.H.Carney,M.G.Guccion and S.B.Baylin(1981).Small cell
carcinoma of the lung: cellular origin and relationship to other
pulmonary tumors. In F.A.Greco,R.K.Oldham,P.A.Bunn Jr.(Eds.),Small
cell lung cancer. Orlando,Fla, Grune & Stratton,pp.145-176.

Gazdar,A.F.(1984).Endocrine tumors of the lung:biology. In K.Becker
and A.F.Gazdar(Eds.), The Endocrine lung in health and disease.
Philadelphia, Saunders,p. 546

Gazdar,A.F.,D.H.Carney and J.D.Minna(1984). Biologia del cancro "non
a piccole cellule". Oncologia clinica,10,3-32.

Gazdar,A.F.(1986). The pathology and biology of small cell carcinoma
of the lung. Istocitopatologia,8,151-158.

Gould,V.E.,R.I.Linnoila,V.A.Memoli and co-workers(1983). Neuroendocrine components of bronchopulmonary tract: hiperplasia, dysplasia
and neoplasm. Lab.Invest.,49,519-537.

Hansen,H.H.,P.Dombernosky,M.Hansen and co-workers(1978).Chemothera-
py of advanced smallcell anaplastic carcinoma: superiority in a
randomized trial of 4 drug combination to 3 drug combination. Amm.
Intern.Med.,89,177-181.

Hattori,S.,M.Matsudu,R.Iateishi and co-workers(1972). Oat-cell carcinoma of the lung:its origin and relationship to bronchial carcinoid. Cancer,30,1014-1024.

Kameya,T.,T.Kodama and Y.Shimosato(1982). Ultrastructure of small
cell carcinoma of the lung (oat and intermediate type) in relation
to histogenesis and to carcinoid tumor. In Shimosato Y.,M.R.Mela-
med and P.Nehesheim(Eds.), Morphogenesis of lung cancer,vol.2,Boca
Raton,FL,CRC Press,p.15-44.

Kasurinen,Y. and K.Y.Syrjänen(1986). Peptide hormone immunoreactivity and prognosis in small cell carcinoma of the lung. Respiration,
49,61-67.

Lehto,V.P.,M.Miettinen,D.Dahl and co-workers(1984). Bronchial carcinoid cells containing neural-type intermediate filaments. Cancer,
54,624-628.

Little,C.D.,M.M.Nan,D.N.Carney and co-workers(1983). Amplification
and expression of c-myc oncogene in human lung cancer cell lines.
Nature,306,194-196.

Matthews,M.J.(1979). Effects of therapy onthe behavior and morphology of small cell carcinoma of the lung. Prog.Can.Res.Ther.,11,155-
165.

Matthews,M.J. and Gazdar A.F.(1982). Small cell carcinoma of the lung:
its morphology, behavior and nature. In Y.Shimosato,M.R.Melamed and
P.Nettesheim(Eds.),Morphogenesis of lung cancer,vol.II,Boca Raton,
FL,CRC Press, p.1.

Nomori,H.,Y.Shimasato,S.Morinaga,T.Nakajima and S.Watanabe(1986).
Subtypes of small cell carcinoma of the lung: morphometric, ultrastructure and immunohistochemical analysis. Hum.Pathol.,17,604-613.

Paladugu,R.R.,J.R.Benfield,H.Y.Pak,R.K.Ross and R.L.Teplitz(1985).
Bronchopulmonary Kulchitzky cell carcinomas. A new classification
scheme for typical and atypical carcinoids. Cancer,55,1303-1311.
Radice, P.A.,M.J.Matthews,D.K.Ihde and co-workers(1982). The clini-
cal behavior of a "mixed" small cell/large cell broncogenic car-
cinoma compared to "pure" small cell subtypes. Cancer,50,2894-2902.
Tamai,S.,T.Kameya,K.Yamaguchi and co-workers(1983). Peripheral lung
carcinoid tumor producing predominantly gastrin-releating peptide
(GRP):morphologic and hormonal studies. Cancer,52,273-281.
Wick,M.R.,B.W.Scheithauer and K.Kovacs(1983). Neuron-specific enola-
se in neuroendocrine tumors of the thymus, bronchus and skin. Am.
J.Clin.Path.,79,703-707.
Whang-Peng,J.,C.S.Kao-Shan,E.C.Lee and co-workers(1982). Specific
chromosome defect associated with human small-cell lung cancer.
Science,215,181-182.
Whitwell,F.(1955). Tumorlets of the lung. J.Path.Bart.,70,529-541.
Yang,K.,T.Ulich,I.Tayolr and co-workers(1983). Pulmonary carcinoids:
immunohistochemical demonstration of brain-gut peptides. Cancer,
52,819-823.
Yesner,R.,O.Auerbach and B.Gerste.(1979). Evolution of small cell
lung carcinoma. Chest.,76,360-363.
Yesner,R.(1985). Large cell carcinoma of the lung. Seminars in Dia-
gnostic Pathology,2,255-269.
Yesner,R.(1986). Personal comunication.

Bombesin: From Frog to Small Cell Lung Camcer

Roberto de Castiglione

Farmitalia Carlo Erba S.p.A., Research & Development,
Via dei Gracchi 35, 20146 Milano, Italy

ABSTRACT

The history of bombesin, from its discovery in the skin of the European discoglossid frog *Bombina bombina* up to its possible role as autocrine growth factor
for human small-cell lung carcinoma, is outlined. Attention has been given to
phylogenetic considerations, structure-activity relationships, receptor specificity and biological functions.

KEYWORDS

Autocrine stimulation; biological activity; bombesin; bombesin analogues; bombesin
receptors; frog skin peptides; phylogenesis; small-cell lung cancer; structural
requirements.

INTRODUCTION

The renewed interest in bombesin, a frog skin tetradecapeptide of formula Glp-
$Gln-Arg-Leu-Gly-Asn-Gln-Trp-Ala-Val-Gly-His-Leu-Met-NH_2$, arose a few years ago
when a human analogue was presumed to be an autocrine growth factor for small-cell
lung carcinoma (SCLC) (Moody and others, 1981; Cuttitta and others, 1985).
Object of this paper is to briefly review the history of bombesin and related peptides beginning from their discovery in different animal tissues up to their possible role in the development of this highly malignant tumour.
The discovery of bombesin in 1970 (Anastasi and others, 1971) was another achievement of the long and fruitful collaboration between Vittorio Erspamer, at that
time director of the Institute of Medical Pharmacology I of the University of Rome,
and the Farmitalia Laboratories for Basic Research in Milan. Before then, the
pioneering work of Erspamer in the search for non-mammalian peptides had already
resulted in important contributions in the understanding of the physiological role
of analogous peptides in mammals and in anticipating their structural requirements.
This was the case of eledoisin and physalaemin with regard to substance P, a peptide known for some of its biological effects since 1931 (Euler and Gaddum, 1931),
but reproduced by synthesis (Tregear and others, 1971), and therefore available
for extensive pharmacological studies, only after its characterization from bovine
hypothalamus in 1971 (Chang and others, 1971), years after eledoisin (Sandrin and
Boissonnas, 1962) and physalaemin (Bernardi and others, 1964) have been synthesized.

These two tachykinins -so named by Erspamer himself as opposed to the group of the slow-acting kinins, the bradykinins (Erspamer and Anastasi, 1966)- were originally isolated (and sequenced) from methanol extracts of the posterior salivary glands of the Mediterranean octopodes *Eledone moschata* and *Eledone aldrovandi* (Erspamer and Anastasi, 1962) and, respectively, from methanol extracts of the skin of the South American frog *Phyllomedusa bigilonigerus (Ph. fuscumaculatus)* (Erspamer and others, 1964). (Incidentally, the serendipitous discovery of physalaemin shifted Erspamer's interest from sea invertebrates to amphibians, whose skins proved to be a very rich and apparently inexhaustible source of new peptide structures).

Another example was the amphibian peptide caerulein, considered the common precursor from which both the mammalian hormones gastrin and cholecystokinin (CCK) have evolved (Larsson and Rehfeld, 1977). Ceruletide (international non-proprietary name proposed by the World Health Organization for caerulein) was identified (and sequenced) in the methanol extracts of the skin of the Australian hylid frog *Litoria (Hyla)caerulea* (Anastasi and others, 1967) and synthesized (Bernardi and others, 1967) a year before the partial sequence of CCK was published (Jorpes, 1968). The synthesis of a series of ceruletide analogues made it possible to anticipate the understanding of the crucial role of the sulphated tyrosine residue -both in terms of presence and location (Anastasi and others, 1968)- for the biological pattern of activity of the two mammalian peptide hormones.

When bombesin and alytesin, two structurally and biologically very similar tetradecapeptides, were discovered in 1970 in the methanol extracts of the skin of the European discoglossid frogs *Bombina bombina, Bombina variegata* and *Alytes obstetricans,* respectively (Anastasi and others, 1971), no mammalian counterparts were known. Bombesin, since it was available from the beginning by chemical synthesis (Bernardi and others, 1971), soon gained popularity over alytesin for its astonishing variety of biological effects both on peripheral tissues and on central nervous system functions.

BOMBESIN-LIKE PEPTIDES

At the time of the discovery of bombesin the concept of the "skin-brain-gut triangle" (Erspamer and Melchiorri, 1980) had not yet been formally established. (This concept, based on embryogenic considerations, states that the same peptides can occur in the skin, brain and gut of vertebrates and, in particular, that peptides present in the skin of amphibians usually have their counterparts in the brain and gut of mammals). Nevertheless, in consideration of the many biological effects displayed by bombesin in experimental animals, it seemed unlikely that the distribution of this or related peptides was restricted only to the frog skin. This consideration eventually led to the identification of bombesin-like immunoreactivity also in amphibian brain (Walsh and others, 1982) and in the brain and gastrointestinal tract of fish (Holmgren and others, 1982; Holmgren and Nilsson, 1983), birds and mammals (Walsh and others, 1979; Melchiorri, 1980), suggesting an evolutionary conservation. The successful structure identification of a bombesin-like peptide from porcine non-antral gastric tissue (Mc Donald and others, 1979), definitely confirmed this assumption. Based on the bioassay used for its isolation, this peptide was given the (misleading) name of gastrin-releasing peptide (GRP).

The search for mammalian bombesin duplicates has recently culminated in the complete sequence determination of human GRP by the complementary efforts of two independently acting research groups. In both cases the source was a hepatic meta-

stasis of a pulmonary carcinoid tumour rich in bombesin-like immunoreactivity.
The approaches were based on cloned cDNA derived from polyadenylated RNA (Spindel
and others, 1984) and on the (partial) microsequence analysis of the isolated
peptide (Orloff and others, 1984).

STRUCTURES AND STRUCTURAL REQUIREMENTS

A complete and updated list of the known structures of bombesin-like peptides is
reported in Table 1. The list includes 16 peptides from amphibians, birds and
mammals. Amino acid residues common to bombesin are in italic.
The major variations are found in the amino-terminal positions of these molecules.
The carboxyl-terminal heptapeptide sequence is highly conserved, with variations
only in position 2 and 5 (counting, unconventionally, from the carboxyl-terminus).
The two phyllolitorins are an exception, having also histidine in the last but two
position replaced by serine. The leucine and phenylalanine residues in penultima-
te position characterize two main peptide groups: the bombesin/GRP and the litorin
(ranatensin)/neuromedin subfamilies, respectively. In position 5 the first group
accepts only valine, whereas the second can accommodate either valine or threonine.
Testing of a series of synthetic bombesin fragments on a battery of *in vitro* smooth
muscle systems (Broccardo and others, 1975) revealed that the carboxyl-terminal
nonapeptide of the parent compound is required for full biological activity. The
carboxyl-terminal hepta- and octapeptides retain some activity, whereas shorter
fragments or amino-terminal sequences are completely inactive (Table 2).
The importance of this region for biological activity was confirmed also in *in vivo*
experiments. Carboxyl-terminal fragments longer than the heptapeptide are effective gastrin releasers in the dog (Sopranzi and Melchiorri, 1973). Alterations
in the carboxyl-terminal tripeptide (such as deletion of the histidine or of the
last two amino acid residues, and oxidation or deamidation of the terminal methio-
nine), as well as inversion of configuration of single amino acid residues in the
carboxyl-terminal heptapeptide, drastically reduce central hypothermic effects in
the rat. The glycine residue, however, can be replaced by D-alanine with full
retention of activity, but not by other amino acid residues of either configuration
(Rivier and Brown, 1978; Moody and others, 1982) (Table 3).
The highly conserved carboxyl-terminal region is essential also for high affinity
binding activity to CNS neurons (Moody and others, 1978), dispersed pancreatic
acini (Jensen and others, 1978), pituitary cells (Westendorf and Schonbrunn, 1983)
and SCLC cells (Moody and others, 1985). Alterations in the amino-terminal region
are of minor importance: bombesin and alytesin are equipotent (Broccardo and others,
1975) and both bombesin and the heptacosapeptide GRP can induce similar biological
responses (Brown and others, 1980; Rockaeus and others, 1982; Girard and others,
1983; Mc Donald and others, 1983).

OCCURRENCE OF BOMBESIN-LIKE IMMUNOREACTIVITY IN HUMANS

In humans, bombesin/GRP-like immunoreactivity has been identified in the lung
(Wharton and others, 1978; Cutz and others, 1981; Johnson and others, 1982; Price
and others, 1983; Tutsumi and others, 1983), stomach (Tobe and others, 1982), pancreas (Ghatei and others, 1984), pituitary (Major and others, 1983), cerebrospinal
fluid (Yamada and others, 1981) and plasma (Wood and others, 1981).
In the lung, the immunoreactivity has been localized both in single neuroendocrine
cells ("APUD" cells) and in groups of these cells called neuro-epithelial bodies.
In fetal lung bombesin-like immunoreactive cells are found at all levels of the

TABLE 1. STRUCTURE OF NATURALLY OCCURRING BOMBESIN-LIKE PEPTIDES.

PEPTIDE	Length of sequence	AMINO ACID SEQUENCE
AMPHIBIANS		
Bombesin [a]	14	Glp-Gln-Arg-Leu-Gly-Asn-Gln-Trp-Ala-Val-Gly-His-Leu-Met-NH_2
Alytesin [a]	14	Glp-Gly-Arg-Leu-Gly-Thr-Gln-Trp-Ala-Val-Gly-His-Leu-Met-NH_2
Litorin [b]	9	Glp-Gln-Trp-Ala-Val-Gly-His-Phe-Met-NH_2
[Glu(OMe)^2]-litorin [c]	9	Glp-Glu(OMe)-Trp-Ala-Val-Gly-His-Phe-Met-NH_2
[Glu(OEt)^2]-litorin [d]	9	Glp-Glu(OEt)-Trp-Ala-Val-Gly-His-Phe-Met-NH_2
Ranatensin [e]	11	Glp-Val-Pro-Gln-Trp-Ala-Val-Gly-His-Phe-Met-NH_2
Ranatensin-C [f]	11	Glp-Thr-Pro-Gln-Trp-Ala-Val-Gly-His-Phe-Met-NH_2
Ranatensin-R [f]	17	Ser-Asp-Ala-Thr-Leu-Arg-Arg-Tyr-Asn-Gln-Trp-Ala-Thr-Gly-His-Phe-Met-NH_2
[Leu^8]-phyllolitorin [g]	9	Glp-Leu-Trp-Ala-Val-Gly-Ser-Leu-Met-NH_2
Phyllolitorin [g]	9	Glp-Leu-Trp-Ala-Val-Gly-Ser-Phe-Met-NH_2
Rohdei-litorin [h]	9	Glp-Leu-Trp-Ala-Thr-Gly-His-Phe-Met-NH_2
BIRDS		
Chicken GRP [i]	27	Ala-Pro-Leu-Gln-Pro-Gly-Gly-Ser-Pro-Ala-Leu-Thr-Lys-Ile-Tyr-Pro-Arg-Gly-Ser-His-Trp-Ala-Val-Gly-His-Leu-Met-NH_2
MAMMALS		
Canine GRP [j]	27	Ala-Pro-Val-Pro-Gly-Gly-Gln-Gly-Thr-Val-Leu-Asp-Lys-Met-Tyr-Pro-Arg-Gly-Asn-His-Trp-Ala-Val-Gly-His-Leu-Met-NH_2
Porcine GRP [k]	27	Ala-Pro-Val-Ser-Val-Gly-Gly-Gly-Thr-Val-Leu-Ala-Lys-Met-Tyr-Pro-Arg-Gly-Asn-His-Trp-Ala-Val-Gly-His-Leu-Met-NH_2
Human GRP [l,m]	27	Val-Pro-Leu-Pro-Ala-Gly-Gly-Gly-Thr-Val-Leu-Thr-Lys-Met-Tyr-Pro-Arg-Gly-Asn-His-Trp-Ala-Val-Gly-His-Leu-Met-NH_2
Porcine neuromedin B [n]	10	Gly-Asn-Leu-Trp-Ala-Thr-Gly-His-Phe-Met-NH_2

a) Anastasi and others, 1971;   b) Anastasi and others, 1975;   c) Anastasi and others, 1977;   d) Nakajima and others, 1980;

e) Nakajima and others, 1970;   f) Nakajima and others, 1979;   g) Yasuhara and others, 1983;   h) Barra and others, 1985;

i) McDonald and others, 1980;   j) Reeve jr. and others, 1983;   k) McDonald and others, 1979;   l) Orloff and others, 1984;

m) Spindell and others, 1984;   n) Minamino and others, 1983.

TABLE 2. RELATIVE POTENCY OF BOMBESIN FRAGMENTS, ON A WEIGHT BASIS (BOMBESIN= 100) (Broccardo and others, 1975)

PEPTIDE	Rat uterus	Rat urinary bladder	Guinea pig urinary bladder	Guinea pig large intestine	Kitten small intestine	Rat large intestine
Glp-Gln-Arg-Leu-Gly-Asn-Gln-Trp-Ala-Val-Gly-His-Leu-Met-NH$_2$ (bombesin)	100	100	100	100	100	100
His-Leu-Met-NH$_2$	< 0.1 (2)	< 0.1 (3)	-	< 0.1 (2)	0.2 (2)	-
Ala-Val-Gly-His-Leu-Met-NH$_2$	< 0.05 (5)	< 0.01 (2)	0.1-0.2 (2)	< 0.1 (7)	< 0.1 (5)	< 0.1 (3)
Trp-Ala-Val-Gly-His-Leu-Met-NH$_2$	2.5-10 (4)	0.2-0.5 (4)	0.2-0.4 (3)	0.1-0.5 (7)	< 0.1-3 (10)	0.5-1 (3)
Gln-Trp-Ala-Val-Gly-His-Leu-Met-NH$_2$	20-30 (6)	2-10 (4)	2-4 (4)	2-10 (7)	1-4 (17)	10-20 (3)
Asn-Gln-Trp-Ala-Val-Gly-His-Leu-Met-NH$_2$	130-300 (7)	150-300 (4)	200-350 (3)	100-120 (7)	100-150 (11)	90-130 (3)
Gly-Asn-Gln-Trp-Ala-Val-Gly-His-Leu-Met-NH$_2$	150-200 (5)	100-150 (3)	150-200 (3)	110-200 (5)	90-200 (8)	70-90 (3)
Leu-Gly-Asn-Gln-Trp-Ala-Val-Gly-His-Leu-Met-NH$_2$	50-200 (8)	100-170 (5)	200-400 (5)	100-160 (6)	80-150 (8)	90-100 (3)
Glp-Gly-Arg-Leu-Gly-Thr-Gln-Trp *	< 0.01 (2)	< 0.1 (2)	-	< 0.1 (2)	< 0.1 (2)	< 0.1 (2)
Glp-Gly-Arg *	< 0.01 (2)	< 0.1 (2)		< 0.01 (2)	< 0.1 (2)	< 0.1 (2)

The number of experiments is given in parentheses.

*Alytesin partial sequence.

R. de Castiglione

TABLE 3. RELATIVE POTENCY OF BOMBESIN ANALOGOUES   (Rivier and others, 1978; Moody and others, 1982)

P E P T I D E	Relative Potency (*)	IC_{50} nM (**)
Glp-Gln-Arg-Leu-Gly-Asn-Gln-Trp-Ala-Val-Gly-His-Leu-Met-NH₂ (bombesin)	100	15
————————————————————————————NHMe	70	--
————————————————————————————OH	<1	800
——————————————————————Met(O)—	<1	350
——————————————————————met———	10	600
———————————————————□———	10	>5000
———————————————————leu———	<1	>5000
———————————————————Phe———	70	--
——————————————his———	0.1	--
—————————————□————	1	200
————————————————Tyr———	1	1000
———————————Ala——— —	1	--
———————————ala———	100	--
———————————Pro———	1	--
———————————pro———	1	--
————————————val———	1	>5000
——————————ala———	5	--
—————————trp———	1	>5000
————————gln———	100	--
————————gln———ala———	100	--
——————asn———	1	--
——————ala———	100	--
—————Lys———	95	--
—————Tyr———	100	--
————Lys———	100	--
——Gly———Thr———(alytesin)———	100	80
Glp-Val-Pro———(ranatensin)———Phe———	20	60
Glp———(litorin)———Phe———	5	40
———————————	1	--
———————————Phe———	1	--

Identical residues are represented by solid lines, while residues of D-amino acids and deleted amino acids are represented by small letters and open boxes, respectively.

(*) Hypothermia i.c.v.   (**) Inhibition of binding of $\left[^{125}I\text{-}Tyr^4\right]$ bombesin to rat brain membranes.

developing bronchial tree, whereas in post-natal and adult lung they are concentrated mostly in the peripheral airway (Cutz and others, 1981). Bombesin-like
immunoreactivity in the lung is higher in the fetus and just after birth, then
decreases in parallel with the observed decrease in the number of pulmonary neuroendocrine cells (Wharton and others, 1978; Track and Cutz, 1982).
Bombesin/GRP immunoreactivity has been found also in primary lung tumours (Wood
and others, 1981; Yamaguchi and others, 1983; Tamai and others, 1983), with particularly high levels in small-cell carcinomas (Moody and others, 1981; Wood and
others, 1981).
The bombesin-like immunoreactivity in the lung is mainly composed of two molecular
forms: the smaller one predominates in the fetus, whereas both small and large molecular forms are present in equal amount in the adult. The immunoreactivity detected in the small-cell lung carcinoma shows a preponderance of the smaller molecular form. This may be seen as a reversion to a fetal characteristic of the
biosynthetic pathway (Ghatei and others, 1983). On the basis of their molecular
weights (determined in comparison with porcine GRP and bombesin) the larger form
is most probably identifiable with human GRP, while the smaller one could possibly
correspond to the carboxyl-terminal nona- or decapeptide, i.e. GRP_{19-27} or GRP_{18-27}
(Roth and others, 1983; Yoshizaki and others, 1984).
GRP-like immunoreactivity has also been found in two medullary thyroid carcinomas
(Matsubayashi and others, 1984).
Other possible localizations of bombesin-like peptides in humans can be inferred
from results in animals. These include detection of bombesin-like immunoreactivity in rat brain (Brown and others, 1978; Moody and others, 1979), rat and dog
intestine (Walsh and others, 1979; Reeve and others, 1983), feline and porcine
skin (O'Shaughnessy and others, 1983), cow milk (Lazarus and others, 1986) and
experimental rat mammary tumours (Gaudino and others, 1986).

RECEPTORS

Specific, high-affinity bombesin receptors have been found in guinea pig pancreatic
acinar cells (Jensen and others, 1978), rat brain membranes (Moody and others, 1979),
rat pituitary cells (Westendorf and Schonbrunn, 1983), human small-cell lung cancer (Moody and others, 1985), and human pancreatic membranes (Scemama and others,
1986).
On the basis of the dissociation of potency of a series of bombesin-like peptides
in inhibiting the binding of radioiodinated $[Tyr^4]$bombesin, the presence of different bombesin receptor sub-types in various target tissues has been suggested
(Westendorf and Schonbrunn, 1983).
Specific, high-affinity receptors for GRP have been found also in Swiss 3T3 mouse
fibroblast cell lines (Zachary and Rozengurt, 1985). This receptor has been characterized as a cell surface protein of 115 kd with ligand- stimulated tyrosine-
specific protein kinase activity (Cirillo and others, 1986).

BIOLOGICAL ACTIVITY

Although a physiological role for bombesin has not yet been firmly established,
bombesin and bombesin-like peptides have a wide range of pharmacological actions.
As it is not the scope of this paper to enter into details on this particular
topic, which has already been covered by many reviews (Erspamer and Melchiorri,
1973; Bertaccini, 1976; Erspamer, 1980; Melchiorri, 1980; Erspamer and Melchiorri, 1983; Walsh, 1983), only the most important biological effects will be men-

tioned.

At doses which can possibly be considered as physiological, bombesin is a potent stimulant of gastrin release and gastric acid secretion, a potent releaser of CCK and a powerful direct stimulant of gall bladder musculature and pancreatic acini. At relatively higher doses it displays marked effects on the myoeletric and mechanical activity of the gut. Finally, by central administration in the rat, bombesin is the most potent agent acting on thermoregulation, glucoregulation, and prolactin and growth hormone release. Antinociceptive effects, not reversed by naloxone, are also observed.

GROWTH-FACTOR ACTIVITY AND SMALL-CELL LUNG CARCINOMA

In addition to the above-mentioned biological effects, bombesin and related peptides display mitogenic activity both *in vivo* and *in vitro*.

Chronic administration of bombesin to rats induces gastric cell hyperplasia, increased pancreatic DNA and enzyme content and increased pancreas to body weight ratio (Lezoche and others, 1981; Lehy and others, 1983). These effects can be either the result of a direct stimulation of the target cells or the consequence of the release of other hormones, such as gastrin (Delle Fave and others, 1980), CCK (Fender and others, 1976; Miyata and others, 1978) or growth hormone (Rivier and others, 1978; Westendorf and Schonbrunn, 1982; Bicknell and Chapman, 1983). In the human respiratory tract, the observed variations in the number of bombesin-containing cells, which steadily increase during gestation, reach a plateau at birth, then dramatically decrease in the adult, suggest a possible role for bombesin-related peptides in fetal lung development (Johnson and others, 1982; Ghatei and others, 1983).

In vitro bombesin stimulates proliferation of the 3T3 mouse fibroblast line (Rozengurt and Sinnett-Smith, 1982) and human bronchial epithelial cells (Willey and others, 1984). Human SCLC cell lines produce and secrete bombesin-like peptides (Sorenson and others, 1982; Moody and others, 1983a) and can express a single class of high affinity receptors for these peptides (Moody and others, 1983b).

Exogenously added bombesin-like peptides can stimulate the clonal growth and DNA synthesis of SCLC in serum-free medium (Carney and others, 1983). A monoclonal antibody to bombesin (having the antigenic determinant localized at the carboxyl-terminal region of the molecule) blocks the binding of the peptide hormone to cellular receptors and inhibits the clonal growth of SCLC *in vitro* and the growth of SCLC xenograft *in vivo* in nude mice (Cuttitta and others, 1985). Taken together, all these findings strongly support the existence of an autocrine mechanism regulating SCLC proliferation mediated by bombesin-like peptides acting as autocrine growth factors.

CONCLUDING REMARKS

The observed behaviour of bombesin-like peptides during lung development and in small-cell lung carcinoma makes these peptides ideal candidates for the role of "autocrine" growth factors. According to the "autocrine" hypothesis (Sporn and Todaro, 1980), "autocrine" growth factors are hormone-like substances (produced and secreted by normal or malignant cells) which induce proliferation of these same cells through activation of specific membrane receptors. This "autocrine" mechanism for self-stimulation, which confers obvious selective growth advantages on very early embryonic cells and can help to account for the explosive growth and multiplication of cells during the earliest stages of the embryogenesis, is poten-

tially very dangerous to the survival of the organism if it is not closely regulated as soon as it is no longer used (Todaro and others, 1981).
The possibility of interfering with this "autocrine" pathway in the case of the small-cell lung carcinoma has already been demonstrated with a monoclonal antibody to bombesin. Another way to block the growth of this tumour is by competing for the bombesin receptors with highly potent and selective bombesin-antagonists. At present, different research groups, including ourselves, are actively working in this direction.

REFERENCES

Anastasi, A., L. Bernardi, G. Bertaccini, G. Bosisio, R. de Castiglione, V. Erspamer, O. Goffredo, and O. Impicciatore (1968). Synthetic peptides related to caerulein. Note I. *Experientia*, 24, 771-773.

Anastasi, A., V. Erspamer, and R. Endean (1967). Isolation and structure of caerulein, an active decapeptide from the skin of *Hyla caerulea*. *Experientia*, 23, 699-700.

Anastasi, A., V. Erspamer, and M. Bucci (1971). Isolation and structure of bombesin and alytesin, two analogous active peptides from the skin of the European amphibian *Bombina* and *Alytes*. *Experientia*, 27, 166-167.

Anastasi, A., V. Erspamer, and R. Endean (1975). Amino acid composition and sequence of litorin, a bombesin-like nonapeptide from the skin of the Australian leptodactylid frog *Litoria aurea*. *Experientia*, 31, 510.

Anastasi, A., P. Montecucchi, F. Angelucci, V. Erspamer, and R. Endean (1977). Glu(OMe)[2]-litorin, the second bombesin-like peptide occurring in methanol extracts of the skin of the Australian frog *Litoria aurea*. *Experientia*, 33, 1289.

Barra, D., G. Falconieri Erspamer, M. Simmaco, F. Bossa, P. Melchiorri, and V. Erspamer (1985). Rohdei-litorin: a new peptide from the skin of *Phyllomedusa rohdei*. *FEBS Lett.*, 182, 53-56.

Bernardi, L., G. Bosisio, R. de Castiglione, and O. Goffredo (1967). Synthesis of caerulein. *Experientia*, 23, 700-701.

Bernardi, L., G. Bosisio, O. Goffredo, and R. de Castiglione (1964). Synthesis of physalaemin. *Experientia*, 20, 490-492.

Bernardi, L., R. de Castiglione, O. Goffredo, and F. Angelucci (1971). Synthesis of bombesin. *Experientia*, 27, 873-874.

Bertaccini, G. (1976). Active polypeptides of nonmammalian origin. *Pharmacol. Rev.*, 28, 127-177.

Bicknell, R. J., and C. Chapman (1983). Bombesin stimulates growth hormone secretion from cultured bovine pituitary cells. *Neuroendocrinology*, 36, 33-38.

Broccardo, M., C. Falconieri Erspamer, P. Melchiorri, L. Negri, and R. de Castiglione (1975). Relative potency of bombesin-like peptides. *Br. J. Pharmac.*, 55, 221-227.

Brown, M., R. Allen, J. Villareal, J. Rivier, and W. Vale (1978). Bombesin-like activity: radioimmunologic assessment in biological tissues. *Life Sci.*, 23, 2721-2728.

Brown, M., W. Märki, and J. Rivier (1980). Is gastrin releasing peptide mammalian bombesin? *Life Sci.*, 27, 125-128.

Carney, D. N., H. Oie, T. W. Moody, A. Gazdar, F. Cuttitta, and J. Minna (1983). Bombesin: an autocrine growth factor for human small cell lung cancer cell lines. *Clin. Res.*, 31, 404 [Abstract].

Chang, M. M., S. E. Leeman, and H. D. Niall (1971). Amino acid sequence of substance P. *Nature New Biol.*, 232, 86-87.

Cirillo, D. M., G. Gaudino, L. Naldini, and P. M. Comoglio (1986). Receptor for bombesin with associated tyrosine kinase activity. *Mol. Cell. Biol.*, 6, 4641-4649.

Cuttitta, F., D. J. Carney, J. Mulshine, T. W. Moody, J. Fedorko, A. Fischler, and J. D. Minna (1985). Bombesin-like peptides can function as autocrine growth factors in human small-cell lung cancer. *Nature*, 316, 823-826.

Cutz, E., W. Chan, and N. S. Track (1981). Bombesin, calcitonin and Leu-enkephalin immunoreactivity in endocrine cells of human lung. *Experientia*, 37, 765-767.

Delle Fave, G., A. Kohn, L. de Magistris, M. Mancuso, and C. Sparvoli (1980). Effect of bombesin-stimulated gastrin on gastric acid secretion in man. *Life Sci.*, 27, 993-999.

Erspamer, V. (1980). Peptides of the amphibian skin active on the gut. II. Bombesin-like peptides: isolation, structure, and basic function. In G. B. J. Glass (*)(Ed.), *Gastrointestinal Hormones*. Raven Press, New York. pp. 343-361.

Erspamer, V., and A. Anastasi (1966). Polypeptides active on plain muscle in the amphibian skin. In E.G. Erdös, N. Back, F. Sicuteri, and A. F. Wilde (Eds.), *Hypotensive Peptides*. Springer Verlarg, Berlin. pp. 63-75.

Erspamer, V., A. Anastasi, G. Bertaccini, and J. M. Cei (1964). Structure and pharmacological actions of physalaemin, the main active polypeptide of the skin of *Physalaemus fuscumaculatus*. *Experientia*, 20, 489-490.

Erspamer, V., and P. Melchiorri (1973). Active polypeptides of the amphibian skin and their synthetic analogues. *Pure Appl. Chem.*, 35, 463-494.

Erspamer, V., and P. Melchiorri (1980). Active polypeptides: from amphibian skin to gastrointestinal tract and brain of mammals. *TIPS*, 391-395.

Erspamer, V., and P. Melchiorri (1983). Actions of amphibian skin peptides on the central nervous system and the anterior pituitary. In E. E. Müller and R. M. Mac Leod (Eds.), *Neuroendocrine Perspectives*, Vol. 2. Elsevier Science Publ. B.V., pp. 37-106.

von Euler, U. S., and J. H. Gaddum (1931). An unidentified depressor substance in certain tissue extracts. *J. Physiol. (London)*, 72, 74-87.

Fender, H. R., P. J. Curtis, P. L. Rayford, and J. C. Thompson (1976). Effect of bombesin on serum gastrin and cholecystokinin in dogs. *Surgical Forum*, 37, 414-416.

Gaudino, G., M. De Bortoli, and L. H. Lazarus (1986). A bombesin-related peptide in experimental mammary tumors in rats. In A. Angeli, H. L. Bradlow, and L. Dogliotti (Eds.), *Endocrinology of the Breast: Basic and Clinical Aspects*, Vol. 464. The New York Academy of Sciences, New York. pp. 450-453.

Ghatei, M. A., M. N. Sheppard, S. Henzen-Logman, M. A. Blank, J. M. Polak, and S. R. Bloom (1983). Bombesin and vasoactive intestinal polypeptide in the developing lung: marked changes in acute respiratory distress syndrome. *J. Clin. Endocr. Metab.*, 57, 1226-1232.

Girard, F., C. Aube, S. St—Pierre, and F. B. Joliecoeur (1983). Structure activity studies on neurobehavioural effects of bombesin (BB) and gastrin releasing peptide (GRP). *Neuropeptides*, 3, 443-452.

Holmgren, S., and S. Nilsson (1983). Bombesin-, gastrin/CCK-, 5-hydroxytryptamine-, neurotensin-, somatostatin-, and VIP-like immunoreactivity and catecholamine fluorescence in the gut of the elasmobranch *Squalus acanthias*. *Cell Tissue Res.*, 234, 595-618.

Holmgren, S., C. Vaillant, and R. Dimaline (1982). VIP-, substance P-, gastrin /CCK-, bombesin-, somatostatin- and glucagon-like immunoreactivities in the gut of the rainbow trout, *Salmo gairdneri*. *Cell Tissue Res.*, 223, 142-153.

Jensen, R. T., T. Moody, C. Pert, J. E. Rivier, and J. D. Gardner (1978). Interaction of bombesin and litorin with specific membrane receptors on pancreatic
acinar cells. *Proc. Natl. Acad. Sci. USA,* 75, 6139-6143.

Johnson, D. E., J. E. Lock, R.P. Elde, and T. R. Thomson (1982). Pulmonary neuroendocrine cells in hyaline membrane disease and bronchopulmonary dysplasia.
Pediatric Res., 16, 446-454.

Jorpes, J. E. (1968). The isolation and chemistry of secretin and cholecystokinin.
Gastroenterology, 55, 157-164.

Larsson, L-J., and J. F. Rehfeld (1977). Evidence for a common evolutionary origin
of gastrin and cholecystokinin. *Nature,* 269, 335-338.

Lazarus, L. H., G. Gaudino, W. E. Wilson, and V. Erspamer (1986). An immunoreactive
peptide in milk contains bombesin-like bioactivity. *Experientia,* 42, 822-823.

Lehy, T., J. P. Accary, D. Labeille, and M. Dubrasquet (1983). Chronic administration of bombesin stimulated antral gastrin cell proliferation in the rat. *Gastroenterology,* 84, 914-919.

Lezoche, E., N. Basso, and V. Speranza (1981). Action of bombesin in man. In S. R.
Bloom, and J. M. Polak (Eds.), *Gut Hormones.* Churchill Livingston, London.
pp. 419-424.

Major, J., M. A. Ghatei, and S. R. Bloom (1983). Bombesin-like immunoreactivity
in the pituitary gland. *Experientia,* 39, 1158-1159.

Matsubayashi, S., C. Yanaihara, M. Ohkubo, S. Fukata, Y. Hayashi, H. Tamai, T. Na-
kagawa, A. Miyauchi, K. Kuma, K. Abe, T. Suzuki, and N. Yanaihara (1984).
Gastrin-releasing peptide immunoreactivity in medullary thyroid carcinoma.
Cancer, 53, 2472-2477.

Mc Donald, T. J., M. A. Ghatei, S. R. Bloom, T. E. Adrian, T. Mochizuchi, C. Yanahiara, and N. Yanahiara (1983). Dose-response comparison of canine plasma gastro-
entero-pancreatic hormone responses to bombesin and the porcine gastrin-releasing
peptide (GRP). *Regulat. Peptides,* 5, 125-137.

Mc Donald, T. J., H. Jörnvall, M. Ghatei, S. R. Bloom, and V. Mutt (1980). Characterization of an avian gastric (proventricular) peptide having sequence homology
with the porcine gastrin-releasing peptide and the amphibian peptides bombesin
and alytesin. *FEBS Lett.,* 122, 45-48.

Mc Donald, T. J., H. Jörnvall, G. Nilsson, M. Vagne, M. Ghatei, S. R. Bloom, and
V. Mutt (1979). Characterization of a gastrin releasing peptide from porcine
non-antral gastric tissue. *Biochem. Biophys. Res. Commun.,* 90, 227-233.

Melchiorri, P. (1980). Bombesin-like peptide activity in the gastrointestinal tract
of mammals and birds. In G. B. J. Glass (Ed.), *Gastrointestinal Hormones.* Raven
Press, New York. pp. 717-725.

Minamino, N., K. Kangawa, and H. Matsuo (1983). Neuromedin B: a novel bombesin
-like peptide identified in porcine spinal cord. *Biochem. Biophys. Res. Commun.,*
114, 541-548.

Miyata, M., S. Guzman, P. L. Rayford, and J. C. Thompson (1978). Effect of bombesin
on release of gastrin, CCK and pancreatic exocrine secretion. *Gastroenterology,*
74, part 2, 1173.

Moody, T. W., V. Bertness, and D. N. Carney (1983b). Bombesin like peptides and
receptors in human tumor cell lines. *Peptides,* 4, 683-686.

Moody, T. W., D. N. Carney, F. Cuttitta, K. Quattrocchi, and J. Minna (1985). High
affinity receptors for bombesin/GRP-like peptides on human small cell lung cancer.
Life Sci., 37, 105-113.

Moody, T. W., J. N. Crawley, and R. T. Jensen (1982). Pharmacology and neurochemi-
stry of bombesin-like peptides. *Peptides,* 3, 559-563.

Moody, T. W., and C. B. Pert (1979). Bombesin-like peptides in rat brain: quanti-
tation and biochemical characterization. *Biochem. Biophys. Res. Commun.*, 90,
7-14.

Moody, T. W., C. B. Pert, A. F. Gazdar, D. N. Carney, and J. D. Minna (1981).
High levels of intracellular bombesin characterize human small-cell lung carcinoma. *Science*, 214, 1246-1248.

Moody, T. W., C. B. Pert, J. Rivier, and M. R. Brown (1978). Bombesin: specific
binding to rat brain membranes. *Proc. Natl. Acad. Sci. USA*, 75, 5372-5376.

Moody, T. W., E. K. Russell, T. L. O'Donohue, C. D. Linden, and A. F. Gazdar (1983a).
Bombesin-like peptides in small cell lung cancer: biochemical characterization
and secretion from a cell line. *Life Sci.*, 32, 487-493.

Nakajima, T., T. Tanimura, and J. J. Pisano (1970). Isolation and structure of a
new vasoactive polypeptide. *Federation Proc.*, 29, 282.

Nakajima, T., T. Yasuhara, and O. Ishikawa (1979). New frog skin peptides homolo-
gous to the ranatensin and bombesin family. In A. Miyoshi (Ed.), *Gut Peptides -
Secretion, Function and Clinical Aspects*. Elsevier Biomedical Press, Tokyo.
pp. 14-18.

Orloff, M. S., J. R. jr. Reeve, C. M. Ben-Avram, J. E. Shively, and J. H. Walsh
(1974). Isolation and sequence analysis of human bombesin-like peptides.
Peptides, 5, 865-870.

O'Shaughnessy, D. J., G. P. Mc Gregor, M. A. Ghatei, M. A. Blank, D. R. Springall,
J. Gu, J. M. Polak, and S. R. Bloom (1983). Distribution of bombesin, somatostatin, substance P and vasoactive intestinal polypeptide in feline and porcine
skin. *Life Sci.*, 32, 2827-2836.

Price, J., E. Penman, G. L. Bourne, and L. H. Rees (1983). Characterization of
bombesin-like immunoreactivity in human fetal lung. *Regulat. Peptides*, 7, 315-
322.

Reeve, J. R. jr., J. H. Walsh, P. Chew, B. Clark, D. Hawke, and J. E. Shively
(1983). Amino acid sequences of three bombesin-like peptides from canine intestine extracts. *J. Biol. Chem.*, 258, 5582-5588.

Rivier, J. E., and M. R. Brown (1978). Bombesin, bombesin analogues, and related
peptides: effects on thermoregulation. *Biochemistry*, 17, 1766-1771.

Rivier, C., J. Rivier, and W. Vale (1978). The effect of bombesin and related
peptides on prolactin and growth hormone secretion in the rat. *Endocrinology*,
102, 519-522.

Rockaeus, A., N. Yanaihara, and T. Mc Donald (1982). Increased concentration of
neurotensin-like immunoreactivity (NTLI) in rat plasma after administration of
bombesin and bombesin-like peptides (porcine and chicken gastrin releasing peptides). *Acta Physiol. Scandin.*, 114, 605-610.

Roth, K. A., C. J. Evans, E. Weber, J. D. Barchas, D. G. Bostwick, and K. G.
Bensch(1983). Gastrin-releasing peptide related peptides in a human malignant
lung carcinoid tumor. *Cancer Res.*, 43, 5411-5415.

Rozengurt, E., and J. Sinnett-Smith (1983). Bombesin stimulation of DNA synthesis
and cell division in cultures of Swiss 3T3 cells. *Proc. Natl. Acad. Sci. USA*,
80, 2936-2940.

Sandrin, E., and R. S. Boissonnas (1962). Synthesis of eledoisin. *Experientia*,
18, 59-61.

Scemama, J.-L., A. Zahidi, D. Fourmy, P. Fagot-Revurat, N. Vaysse, L. Pradayrol,
and A. Ribet (1986). Interaction of $[^{125}I]$-Tyr^4-bombesin with specific receptors
on normal human pancreatic membranes. *Regulat. Peptides*, 13, 125-132.

Sopranzi, N., and P. Melchiorri (1973). Natural and synthetic bombesin-like peptides as gastrin releasers. *J. Pharmacol.*, 5, 125.

Soreson, G. D., S. R. Bloom, M. A. Ghatei, S. A. Del Prete, C. C. Cate, and O. S. Pettengill (1982). Bombesin production by human small cell carcinoma of the lung. *Regulat. Peptides, 4*, 59-66.

Spindel, E. R., W. W. Chin, J. Price, L. H. Rees, G. M. Besser, and J. F. Habener (1984). Cloning and characterization of cDNAs encoding human gastrin-releasing peptides. *Proc. Natl. Acad. Sci. USA, 81*, 5699-5703.

Sporn, M. B., and G. J. Todaro (1980). Autocrine secretion and malignant transformation of cells. *New England J. Med., 303*, 878-880.

Tamai, S., T. Kameya, K. Yamaguchi, N. Yanai, K. Abe, N. Yanaihara, H. Yamazaki, and K. Kageyama (1983). Peripheral lung carcinoid tumor producing predominantly gastrin-releasing peptide (GRP). *Cancer, 52*, 272-281.

Tobe, T., A. Yamahiro, T. Manabe, M. Noguchi, K. Okaji, and H. Yajima (1982). Gastrin releasing peptide (GRP) in the human stomach. *Acta Histochem. Cytochem., 15*, 102-107.

Todaro, G. J., J. E. De Larco, C. Fryling, P. A. Johnson, and M. B. Sporn (1981). Transforming growth factors (TGFs): properties and possible mechanisms of action. *J. Supramol. Struct. Cell. Biochem., 15*, 287-301.

Track, N. S., and E. Cutz (1982). Bombesin-like immunoreactivity in developing human lung. *Life Sci., 30*, 1553-1556.

Tregear, G. W., H. D. Niall, J. T. jr. Potts, S. E. Leeman, and M. M. Chang (1971). Synthesis of substance P. *Nature New Biol., 232*, 87-89.

Tutsumi, Y., R. Y. Osamura, K. Watanabe, and N. Yanaihara (1983). Immunohistochemical studies on gastrin-releasing peptide- and adrenocorticotropic hormone- containing cells in human lung. *Lab. Invest., 48*, 623-631.

Walsh, J. H. (1983). Bombesin-like peptides. In D. T. Krieger, M. J. Brownstein, and J. B. Martin (Eds.), *Brain Peptides*. Wiley-Interscience Publ.. pp. 941-960.

Walsh, J. H., J. Lechago, H. C. Wong, and G. L. Rosenquist (1982). Presence of ranatensin-like and bombesin-like peptides in amphibian brains. *Regulat. Peptides, 3*, 1-13.

Walsh, J. H., H. C. Wong, and G. J. Dockray (1979). Bombesin-like peptides in mammals. *Fed. Proc., 38*, 2315-2319.

Westendorf, J. M., and A. Schonbrunn (1982). Bombesin stimulates prolactin and growth hormone release by pituitary cells in culture. *Endocrinology, 110*, 352-358.

Westendorf, J. M., and A. Schonbrunn (1983). Characterization of bombesin receptors in a rat pituitary cell line. *J. Biol. Chem., 258*, 7527-7535.

Wharton, J., J. M. Polak, S. R. Bloom, M. A. Ghatei, E. Solcia, M. R. Brown, and A. G. E. Pearse (1978). Bombesin-like immunoreactivity in the lung. *Nature, 273*, 769-770.

Willey, J. C., J. R. Lechner, and C. C. Harris (1984). Bombesin and the C-terminal tetradecapeptide of gastrin-releasing peptide are growth factors for normal human bronchial epithelial cells. *Exp. Cell. Res., 153*, 245-248.

Wood, S. M., J. R. Wood, M. A. Ghatei, Y. C. Lee, D. O'Shaughnessy, and S. R. Bloom (1981). Bombesin, somatostatin and neurotensin-like immunoreactivity in bronchial carcinoma. *J. Clin. Endocr. Metab., 53*, 1310-1312.

Yamada, T., M. S. Takami, and R. H. Gerner (1981). Bombesin-like immunoreactivity in human cerebrospinal fluid. *Brain Res., 223*, 214-217.

Yamaguchi, K., K. Abe, T. Kameya, I. Adachi, S. Taguchi, K. Otsubo, and N. Yanahiara (1983). Production and molecular size heterogeneity of immunoreactive gastrin-releasing peptide in fetal and adult lungs and primary lung tumors. *Cancer Res., 43*, 3932-3939.

Yasuhara, T., T. Nakajima, K. Nokihara, C. Yanaihara, N. Yanaihara, V. Erspamer, and G. Falconieri Erspamer (1983). Two new frog skin peptides, phyllolitorins, of the bombesin-ranatensin family from *Phyllomedusa sauvagei*. *Biomed. Res.*, 4, 407-412.

Yoshizaki, K., V. de Bock, and S. Solomon (1984). Origin of bombesin-like peptides in human fetal lung. *Life Sci.*, 34, 835-843.

Zachary, I., and E. Rozengurt (1985). High-affinity receptors for peptides of the bombesin family in Swiss 3T3 cells. *Proc. Natl. Acad. Sci. USA*, 82, 7616-7620.

(*) Erspamer, V., and A. Anastasi (1962). Structure and pharmacological actions of eledoisin, the active endecapeptide of the posterior salivary gland of *Eledone*. *Experientia*, 20, 489-490.

Lung Cancer and Biology

Desmond N. Carney

Department of Medical Oncology, Mater Hospital, Eccles
Street, Dublic 7, Ireland

ABSTRACT

Lung cancer accounts for the greatest percentage of cancer deaths among males and
females. While considerable advances in therapy have been achieved in the past
decade, the overall results remain poor with 5 year survivals ranging from 5-10%.
Recent studies of established cell lines of both small cell and non-small cell
lung cancer have revealed that considerable heterogeneity exists in the biological properties both between SCLC and NSCLC; and among cell lines of SCLC.
This heterogeneity exists in growth properties, biomarker expression, radiation
sensitivity and oncogene expression. When correlated with clinical studies of
SCLC, the biological properties of tumour cells appear to be of prognostic
importance. Future clinical trials should evaluate the inherent properties of
tumour cells as markers of sensitivity to therapy and survival.

KEYWORDS

Cell lines; defined culture media; biomarkers; antigen expression; oncogenes;
autocrine growth factors.

INTRODUCTION

Lung cancer remains the number one cancer killer in the western world. In 1987
150,000 new cases of lung cancer will be diagnosed in the United States and 130,
000 people will die from this disease. Overall lung cancer accounts for approximately 34% of all cancer deaths in males and 20% of cancer deaths in females.
This year for the first time death from lung cancer will exceed death from breast
carcinoma in women. There are four major histological subtypes of lung cancer;
squamous cell carcinoma, adenocarcinoma, large cell carcinoma (these three collect-
ively referred to as non small cell lung cancer [NSCLC]) and small cell carcinoma
of the lung [SCLC] which accounts for 25% of all new cases of lung cancer. For
patients with NSCLC hope for long term survival and cure is directly related to
the ability to surgically resect this tumour type. NSCLC rarely responds, or
responds poorly, to cytotoxic therapy. In contrast for patients with SCLC hope
for their long term survival is directly related to the sensitivity of this
tumour to combination chemotherapy with or without radiation therapy. While the
majority of patients with SCLC will respond to cytotoxic therapy less than 10% of
all patients will be cured of their disease.

Many factors may influence the response to therapy and survival of patients with
lung cancer including performance status, extent of disease, and metastatic spread
of disease to certain sites such as bone marrow, liver or C.N.S. However it is
also likely that factors inherent to the tumour cells themselves may be of

prognostic importance. In recent years considerable advances in understanding
the biology of lung cancer have been gained by the establishment of cell lines of
this tumour. In this chapter techniques used to establish these cell lines will
be discussed and the biological properties of the cell lines will also be discussed. In consideration of the biology of lung cancer several questions will be
asked: 1) can the biological properties of SCLC be used to distinguish small cell
from non small cell lung cancer? 2) Are the biological properties of lung cancer
clinically important? 3) Can an understanding of the biological properties of
lung cancer lead to the development of new therapeutic modalities for this
disease in vivo?

CELL LINES OF LUNG CANCER

In recent years considerable success has been attained in the establishment of
continuous cell lines of lung cancer including both small cell and non small cell.
This success has been achieved predominantly through the use of chemically
defined hormone supplemented medium for growth of these cells. Previous studies
using non-defined serum supplemented medium (SSM) were associated with a success
rate of establishing SCLC cell lines of approximately 10%. The use of chemically
defined medium (HITES) with or without 2.5% SSM has led to successful establishment of permanent cell lines of SCLC from 75% of all tumour containing specimens
(Carney and co-workers,1985). These include specimens obtained from men and
women, treated and untreated patients, and from a variety of organ sites including lung, bone marrow, lymph node, pleural effusions and other surgically
resected specimens. Once established as permanent cell lines these cells can be
successfully cryopreserved, will form tumours in nude mice and colonies in soft
agarose. In a similar manner considerable success has also been achieved in the
establishment of NSCLC cell lines, in particular that of adenocarcinoma of the
lung. The development of a defined medium (ACL-3) for this tumour type has now
led to the successful establishment of cell lines from approximately 33% of all
freshly obtained specimens (Brower and co-workers, 1986), (Table 1).

SCLC cell lines grow predominantly as floating aggregates of tightly to loosely
packed cells, frequently demonstrating areas of central necrosis. In a recent
study of 50 cell lines all but 3 cell lines grew as floating aggregates, the
remainder as attached monolayer cultures. In contrast cell lines of NSCLC predominantly grow as attached monolayer cultures (Carney and co-workers, 1985;
Brower and co-workers, 1986).

Table 1: Growth Factors for SCLC and Non SCLC Cell Lines and
Clinical Specimens

	Small Cell	Non-Small Cell
Medium Designation	Hites	ACL-3
Basal Medium	RPMI 1640	RPMI 1640
Attachment Factors	-	Collagen/Fibronectin
Hydrocortisone	+	+
Insulin	+	+
Transferrin	+	+
Estradiol	+	-
Selenium	+	+
EGF	-	+
Sodium Pyruvate	-	+
Triiodothyronine	-	+

DIFFERENTIAL EXPRESSION OF BIOMARKERS BY SMALL CELL AND NON
SMALL CELL LUNG CANCER

Detailed studies of a large panel of cell lines of both SCLC and NSCLC and other
tumour types for the expression of a variety of biochemical markers and hormones
indicate that a panel of markers can clearly distinguish small cell from non
small cell tumours (Carney and co-workers, 1985; Carney, 1986). Previous studies
which had clearly demonstrated that SCLC cells had neurosecretory granules and
other studies confirming its ability to secrete peptide hormones suggested that
this tumour type would have many of the features of APUD tumours. Studies of
large panels of cell lines have confirmed these data. The vast majority of cell
lines of SCLC have high levels of the key APUD enzyme L-dopa decarboxylase, the
APUD enzyme neuron specific enolase (NSE), the peptide hormone bombesin/GRP and
the BB isozyme of creatine kinase CK-BB (Carney and co-workers, 1985). In contrast these markers are expressed either at very low levels or not at all in cell
lines of NSCLC origin. As will be discussed further exceptions to these
differences do exist. In addition to cell lines, studies of fresh biopsy
specimens of both small cell and NSCLC also clearly demonstrate that the
expression of these four biomarkers can be used to distinguish small cell from
non small cell tumours. This clearly is of value in the analysis of tumours
where the histology is that of an anaplastic tumour and remains unclear.

The expression of markers such as NSE and CK-BB by SCLC tumours has prompted
many studies of the valuation of these biomarkers as serum markers for disease
extent and response to therapy in patients with SCLC (Carney and co-workers,
1982; Johnson and co-workers, 1985; Splinter and co-workers, 1987). In many
studies reported NSE is elevated in the serum in approximately 70% of newly
diagnosed patients with SCLC. In contrast it is detectable in only 10-15% of
patients with NSCLC. For patients with small cell there is an excellent correlation between the presence of elevated serum NSE and tumour burden. Moreover
there is an excellent correlation with the fall in NSE and overall response to
therapy. In studies thus far an elevated NSE was not associated with the disease
in a specific organ site including the C.N.S. Similar studies in determining
serum CK-BB in SCLC patients have demonstrated that it is elevated in approximately 27% of newly diagnosed patients. All of these patients had extensive
stage disease. Moreover in these studies it has clearly been demonstrated that
the presence of an elevated serum CK-BB at diagnosis is an independent poor
prognostic factor for patients with this disease. Further studies have also
evaluated the finding of NSE, CK-BB, bombesin and calcitonin in the C.S.F. as a
marker of metastatic spread to this site in patients with SCLC (Hansen, 1986).
While there is a differential expression of NSE, bombesin and calcitonin for
patients with either cerebral or parenchymal metastases in contrast to patients
with meningeal carcinomatosis, further studies are required to determine if
early detection of these markers in the C.S.F. would be the first indicator of
metastatic disease from SCLC to these metastatic sites.

Considerable heterogeneity has also been noted in the expression of dopa
decarboxylase among cell lines of SCLC (Carney and co-workers, 1985). Among
approximately 70% of all cell lines significantly elevated levels of DDC are
noted. However for the remaining 30% of cell lines either very low levels or
undetectable levels of DDC are noted. Thus the presence or absence of DDC among
cell lines of SCLC allows the subdivision of these cell lines into two major sub-
classes, namely, classic SCLC cell lines with elevated levels of DDC and variant
cell lines with low or undetectable levels. As noted in Table 2 there are other
considerable biological differences in cell lines of these two major types.
Variant cell lines grow as looser floating aggregates of cells, have a higher
cloning efficiency and faster doubling time than classic cell lines, have lower
or undetectable levels of both dopa decarboxylase and bombesin/GRP, lower levels
or neuron specific enolase, but continue to express high levels of CK-BB. This
latter is in marked contrast to that of NSCLC which has undetectable levels of
CK-BB.

Variant cell lines also show marked differences in responses to radiation
therapy and in oncogene expression. Thus there is considerable heterogeneity in
the expression of biomarkers of small cell carcinoma of the lung which appears to
be of major biological importance. Further studies are required to confirm that
these biological differences are of clinical importance.

Table 2: Biological Properties of Lung Cancer Cell Lines

Characteristic	SCLC		Non-SCLC
	Classic	Variant	
Morphology	Float	Float	Attached
Cytology	SCLC	SCLC/LC	NSCLC
DOPA	++	-	-
Bombesin	++	-	-
NSE	++	-	-
CK-BB	++	++	-
Doubling Time	> 2 hr	32 hr	40 hr
Cloning Efficiency	2.6% (1-5)	13.2%	6%
C-myc Amplification	-	+	-
N-myc Amplification	+/-	-	-
L-myc Amplification	+/-	-	-
Chromosome 3p Deletion	+	+	-

IN VITRO RADIATION SENSITIVITY OF LUNG CANCER CELL LINES

Several investigators have reported on the in vitro radiobiological properties of
cell lines of both SCLC and NSCLC. Detailed studies of SCLC have demonstrated
that classic cell lines demonstrate a marked radiation sensitivity in vitro,
typical of what is observed in the clinical situation (Carney, Kinsella, Mitchell,
1983; Morstyn and co-workers, 1984). In contrast variant cell lines demonstrate
a relative radioresistance in vitro. These studies reveal that classic cell lines
have a low extrapolation number $\bar{n}$ ranging from 1.0-3.3. In contrast variant cell
lines have an $\bar{n}$ value ranging from 5.5-11.0, indicating a relative resistance of
these lines to radiation. Moreover at a 200 rad fraction (the dose frequently
used clinically to treat patients with lung cancer) the surviving fraction of
variant cell lines is significantly greater than that of classic cell lines.
These data suggest that if radiation therapy is used to treat patients with the
variant phenotype of SCLC higher single dose fractions may be required to demonstrate a clinical effect. For NSCLC cell lines considerable heterogeneity in the
in vitro radiation survival is observed with wide ranges in both the Do's and
extrapolation number $\bar{n}$.

ONCOGENE EXPRESSION IN SCLC CELLS

Considerable studies have been carried out on the expression of a variety of
oncogenes in both fresh specimens and cell lines of SCLC. The majority of these
studies have clearly demonstrated that increased expression and amplification of
oncogenes of the myc family are expressed in many specimens, in particular cell
lines of SCLC (Little and co-workers, 1983; Nau and co-workers, 1986a; Nau and
co-workers, 1986b). In a recent report of 44 cell lines of SCLC increased
amplification of myc related genes was detected in 44% of such specimens. These
included amplification of C-myc, N-myc and L-myc. The majority of cell lines of
the variant phenotype which were noted to have a significantly faster doubling
rate than that of classic cell lines were amplified for C-myc. Amplification of
N-myc and L-myc was seen more frequently in classic cell lines of SCLC.

In cell lines obtained from patients who had received prior chemotherapy increased amplification of these oncogenes was noted in 44% of specimens. In contrast only 1 specimen or 10% of the cell lines from patients who had not received chemotherapy were amplified for these oncogenes. These data do suggest that the chemotherapy used may be of importance in the ultimate expression of these oncogenes. However when studies of fresh specimens were carried out including 24 specimens obtained from previously treated patients only 3 specimens or 12% were amplified for any of the myc related oncogenes. When one contrasts the data from fresh specimens with that of cell lines there is a suggestion that increased expression and amplification of these oncogenes may in some cases be an artefact of tissue culture. Further studies of greater numbers of fresh specimens are required to determine the relevance of myc oncogene amplification in small cell carcinoma.

ANTIGENIC EXPRESSION IN LUNG CANCER

Numerous studies have reported on antigenic expression and monoclonal antibodies in both small cell and non small cell carcinoma. The vast majority of studies with monoclonal antibodies have suggested that few antibodies are entirely specific for an individual class of lung cancer, i.e., small cell or non small cell carcinoma. In spite of this several clinical studies have been reported on the clinical uses of monoclonal antibodies. Immunohistochemistry studies using the monoclonal antibody SM1 have revealed that up to 50% of bone marrow aspirate specimens from patients with limited stage SCLC, in which routine pathology studies have failed to demonstrate tumour cells, stain positive for tumour cells with this antibody (Stahel and co-workers, 1985). Similar studies have been reported by other investigators. Thus these studies do suggest that the detection of tumour cells may be significantly improved through the use of the panels of monoclonal antibodies. The data will also have a major impact on therapy selection for patients with lung cancer, particularly in the consideration of the uses of autologous bone marrow transplantation. Detailed studies of the expression of the major histocompatibility complex antigens (HLA, A, B, C and B_2 microglobulin) have revealed differential expression of these antigens between small cell and non small cell lung cancer (Doyle and co-workers, 1985). Marked deficiencies of expression of these antigens are observed in small cell carcinoma cell lines in contrast to NSCLC lines, which have been found to readily express these antigens. Moreover the expression of these antigens in SCLC can be modulated and increased by the use of interferons. This has been observed both clinically and in vitro. As differences in the expression of HLA antigens can be observed in fresh biopsies of lung cancer the detection and assessment in fresh biopsies may be of clinical importance in the evaluation of anaplastic tumours. The differential expression of these antigens by small cell and non small cell may also account for some of the biological differences between these two major categories of lung cancer, in particular the early wide spread of disease frequently noted in patients with SCLC.

BOMBESIN AND GROWTH FACTORS FOR SMALL CELL CARCINOMA OF THE LUNG

The ability to culture permanent cell lines of small cell lung cancer in serum free chemically defined medium has greatly facilitated the establishment of cell lines from fresh biopsy specimens. In addition however it has also greatly facilitated the search for specific autocrine growth factors for this tumour type. Initial studies using established cell lines of small cell carcinoma of the lung had clearly demonstrated that condition medium obtained from cells growing in HITES was mitogenic for other tumour cells, suggesting that autocrine growth factors were being secreted for this tumour type. Recent data of characterization of factors in this condition medium suggest that somatomedin/C or insulin like growth factor 1 is one of the major mitogenic factors secreted by small cell

carcinoma of the lung and which may function as an autocrine growth factor
(Macauley and co-workers, 1987).

Bombesin and gastrin releasing peptide have been demonstrated in the vast majority
of cell lines of SCLC in contrast to other cell types of lung cancer. In addition it has been previously demonstrated that bombesin is actively secreted by
these cells into the culture medium and that many cell lines of SCLC have high
affinity binding receptors for this tumour type (Moody, Bertness, Carney, 1983).
All of these data suggest that bombesin/GRP may have an important physiological
role for small cell carcinoma. Studies carried out using an in vitro soft agarose
clonogenic assay have clearly demonstrated that the addition of bombesin results
in up to 150 fold stimulation of the clonal growth of many small cell lung cancer
cell lines (Carney and co-workers, 1987). In contrast bombesin at a similar
concentration has no effect on the clonal growth of a variety of other human
tumour types including NSCLC. In other systems bombesin and GRP are mitogenic for
3T3 mouse fibroblasts, normal human bronchial eipthelial cells in vitro, and in
vivo can cause gastric cell hyperplasia and increased pancreatic DNA content.
These data suggest that bombesin/GRP peptides are important mitogens which in
SCLC may function as autocrine growth factors. Further data confirming this
hypothesis has been the demonstration that a monoclonal antibody 2A11 which
reacts with free bombesin can prevent the growth of SCLC cells both in vitro and
when innoculated into athymic nude mice (Cuttitta and co-workers, 1985). This
monoclonal antibody 2A11 binds to the C-terminal region of bombesin which is that
part of bombesin essential for binding to its receptor of SCLC cells. The
inhibition of growth of small cell lung cancer xenografts in athymic nude mice
suggests that the use of such a monoclonal antibody may be of therapeutic value
in the treatment of patients with this disease.

IS THERE A COMMON STEM CELL FOR ALL CELL TYPES OF LUNG CANCER?

While much data generated in biological studies of cell lines of lung cancer has
clearly demonstrated differences between the major classes, recent areas suggest
that in some circumstances a common stem cell for all types of lung cancer may
exist. Detailed studies of the expression of intermediate cell filaments have
clearly demonstrated that the major ICP in both SCLC and NSCLC are cytokeratins
(Broers and co-workers, 1985; Broers and co-workers, 1986). Moreover studies of
large numbers of cell lines of NSCLC and fresh biopsy specimens have demonstrated
that while these cell lines histologically resemble NSCLC, biochemically in 10-
15% they have many features in common with small cell including expression of
high levels of dopa decarboxylase, bombesin and NSE. In vitro studies on two cell
lines derived from patients with SCLC have clearly demonstrated the ability of
these cell lines to undergo tripartite differentiation in vitro into small cell,
squamous cell and adenocarcinoma of the lung. Taken together these data suggest
an overlap in the expression of biological properties and biochemical markers by
small cell and non small cell carcinoma. As some clinical data suggests that the
endocrine properties of small cell carcinoma of the lung may be important in
predicting responses to therapy and survival, consideration should be given to
the characterization of lung carcinoma as endocrine and non endocrine tumours
based on the expression of dopa decarboxylase in the assessment of clinical trials
in the future. Further data supporting this has been the demonstration that
patients from whom variant cell lines of SCLC are derived, i.e., non endocrine
small cell carcinoma tumours, have a significantly poorer response to therapy and
survival than patients with the classic phenotype.

SUMMARY

Considerable advances in understanding the biology of lung cancer have been made
in recent years. Detailed studies reveal that heterogeneity does exist both in
small cell and non small cell carcinoma of the lung.

Many markers will help distinguish between the two major classes of lung carcinoma. However as considerable overlap does exist future clinical trials should examine the expression of biomarkers in fresh biopsy specimens to determine if these indeed are important in predicting responses to therapy and overall survival for patients with these diseases.

REFERENCES

Carney, D.N., A.F. Gazdar, G. Bepler, J. Guccion, T.W. Moody, P.J. Marangos, M.H. Zweig, and J.D. Minna (1985). Establishment and identification of small cell lung cancer cell lines having classic and variant features. Cancer Res., 45, 2913-2923.

Brower, M., D.N. Carney, H.K. Oie, A.F. Gazdar, and J.D. Minna (1986). Growth of cell lines and clinical specimens of human non-small cell lung cancer in a serum-free defined medium. Cancer Res., 46, 798-806.

Carney, D.N. (1986). Recent advances in the biology of small cell lung cancer. Chest, 89, 4, 253-257.

Carney, D.N., P.J. Marangos, D.C. Ihde, P.A. Bunn, M.H. Cohen, J.D. Minna, and A.F. Gazdar (1982). Serum neuron specific enolase: A marker for disease extent and response to therapy in patients with small cell lung cancer. Lancet, i, 583-585.

Johnson D.H., P.J. Marangos, J.T. Forbes, J.D. Hainsworth, R. Van Welch, and K.R. Hande (1984). Potential utility of serum neuron specific enolase levels in small cell carcinoma of the lung. Cancer Res., 44, 5409.

Cooper E.H., T.A.W. Splinter, and D.A. Brown (1985). Evaluation of a radio-immunoassay for neuron specific enolase in small cell lung cancer. Br. J. Cancer, 52, 333-338.

Hansen, M., and A.G. Pedersen (1986). Tumour markers in patients with lung cancer. Chest, 89, 4, 219-224.

Carney, D.N., J.R. Mitchell, and T.J. Kinsella (1983). In vitro radiation and chemosensitivity of established cell lines of human small cell lung cancer and its large cell variants. Cancer Res., 43, 2806-2811.

Morstyn G., A. Russo, D.N. Carney, E. Karawya, S.H. Wilson, and J. Mitchell (1984). Heterogeneity in the radiation survival curves and biochemical properties of human lung cancer cell lines. J. Natl. Cancer Inst., 801-807.

Little C.D., M.M. Nau, D.N. Carney, A.F. Gazdar, and J.D. Minna (1983). Amplification and expression of the C-myc oncogene in human lung cancer cell lines. Nature, 306, 194-196.

Nau M.M., B.J. Brooks, D.N. Carney, A.F. Gazdar, J.F. Battey, E.A. Sausville and J.D. Minna (1986). Human small cell lung cancer shows amplification and expression of the N-myc gene. Proc. Natl. Acad. Sci. U.S.A., 83, 1092-1096.

Nau M.M., B.J. Brooks, J. Battey, E. Sausville, A.F. Gazdar, I. Kirsch, O.W. McBride, V. Bertness, G.F. Hollis, and J.D. Minna (1986). L-myc, a new myc-related gene amplified and expressed in human cell lung cancer. Nature, 318, 69-72.

Stahel R.A.,   Mambrym, and A.T. Skarin (1985). Detection of bone marrow metastasis in small cell lung cancer by monoclonal antibody. J. Clin. Oncol., 3, 455-461.

Doyle A.F., W.J. Martin, and K. Funa (1985). Marked decreased expression of Class 1 histocompatibility antigens, protein and mRNA in human small cell lung cancer. J. Exp. Med., 161, 1135-1151.

Macauley V., J. Teale, and M. Everard (1987). Somatomedin-C/Insulin like growth factor I is a mitogen for human small cell lung cancer. Proc. Amer. Assoc. Cancer Res., 213.

Moody, T.W., V. Bertness, and D.N. Carney (1983). Bombesin-like peptides and receptors in human tumour cell lines. Peptides, 4, 683-686.

Carney, D.N., F. Cuttitta, T.W. Moody, and J.D. Minna (1987). Selective stimulation of small cell lung cancer clonal growth by bombesin and gastrin-releasing peptide. Cancer Res., 47, 821-825.

Cuttitta F., D.N. Carney, and J. Mulshine (1985). Bombesin-like peptides can
  function as autocrine growth factors in human small cell lung cancer.
  Nature, 316, 823-826.
Broers J.L.V., D.N. Carney, L. de Leij, G.P. Vooijs and F. Ramaekers (1985).
  Differential expression of intermediate filament proteins distinguishes classic
  from variant small cell lung cancer cell lines. Proc. Natl. Acad. Sci., 82,
  4409-4413.
Broers, J.L.V., D.N. Carney, M. Rot Klein, G. Schaart, E.B. Lane, G.P. Vooijs,
  and F.C.S. Ramaekers (1986). Intermediate filament proteins in classic and
  variant types of small cell lung carcinoma cell lines: A biochemical and immuno-
  chemical analysis using a panel of monoclonal and polyclonal antibodies.
  J. Cell Sci., 83, 37-60.

The Biological Bases and Prognostic Factors for a Classification of Small Cell Lung Cancer

Ted Splinter*, Otilia Dalesio[+] and the
EORTC Lung Cancer Group

*University Hospital Dijkzigt, Department of Oncology,
Rotterdam, The Netherlands
[+]EORTC Data Center, Brussels, Belgium

ABSTRACT

The generally acknowledged prognostic factors in small cell lung cancer (SCLC) are extent of disease and performance status. The distinction of extent of disease in limited and extensive disease is a rather crude way to estimate the total body tumour load, which probably is a continuous spectrum from a small peripheral nodule to very extensive involvement of many organs. Recently in several papers it has been shown that biochemical parameters have additional prognostic value, which may be due to the fact that they give a more refined assessment of the extent of disease. In this chapter a short overview of prognostic factors is given. Further the biological bases of possible prognostic factors are discussed and theoretical considerations about a classification are forwarded. Assumptions are made, questions are raised and very few answers are given.

KEYWORDS

small cell lung cancer; classification; prognostic factors; total body tumour mass; tumour doubling time.

INTRODUCTION

It is well known that the results of the treatment of small cell lung cancer (SCLC) have reached a plateau for the last 10 years despite the sensitivity of the tumour for chemotherapy and radiotherapy. In comparison with the V.A. study (Green and others, 1969) the median survival of limited disease (LD) patients has increased from 3 to approx. 14 months and of extensive disease (ED) patients from 1.6 to 10 months. However 90% of all patients will die of their disease within 2 years from start of treatment (Smyth and Hansen, 1985). These figures have not changed despite hundreds of trials, investigating the effect of different chemotherapy- or chemoradiotherapy regimes. Two main trends in the treatment of SCLC can be distinguished. One is directed at improvement of survival by aggressive treatment in an extensively staged selected group of patients. The other is directed at achievement of the present survival with as little burden for the patient as possible, both during staging and treatment. These approaches ask for different staging procedures and classifications.

"OLD" PROGNOSTIC FACTORS

The main and generally accepted consistent prognostic factors for survival in SCLC are performance status and extent of disease (Zelen, 1973). Other less consistent prognostic factors are weight loss; metastases in liver, central nervous system or bone marrow; number of sites of metastases; bulk of the primary tumour; prior radiotherapy and immune status (Ihde, 1985).

It is important to recognize that the more aggressive the staging procedures, such as CT-guided biopsies of the adrenal glands (Pagani, 1983), exploratory laparotomies (Mirra and others, 1981) and bilateral bone marrow punctures (Hirsch and others, 1979) or the more sensitive staging procedures are, such as monoclonal antibodies (Stahel and others, 1985) the higher the percentage of ED patients. This emphasizes the very relative value of the distinction between LD and ED. Most probably the real presentation of SCLC is a continuous spectrum of disease extent from a small peripheral nodule to very extensive involvement of many organs. Patients with LD are more likely to show a superior response rate and survival than ED patients (Maurer and Pajak, 1981). Patients with ED, based on the presence of 1 site of metastasis outside the lung and mediastinum show the same response rate and survival as LD patients (Livingston and others, 1982; Giannone and others, 1987; Jacobs and others, 1980; Maurer and Pajak, 1981; Ihde and others, 1981). The number of sites of metastases in ED patients (Ihde and others, 1981) and the size of the intrathoracic tumour in LD patients (Harper and others, 1982) are strong prognostic factors for response and survival. These data suggest that the total body tumour load is a very important prognostic factor for response and survival in SCLC.

Although little information is available about the reliability and validity of measuring performance status (Orr and Aisner, 1986) in practice PS is of equal or greater prognostic weight than disease stage (Ihde, 1985). Within a given stage PS is an independent predictor of response and survival (Ihde and others, 1981). Even after a complete response was achieved the initial PS exerted an effect on survival (Ihde and others, 1981). Probably PS and extent of disease are often associated, since patients with a worse PS are more likely to have extensive disease (Ihde and others, 1981; Einhorn and others, 1978). However the survival of patients with an impaired PS due to pleural effusion does not seem to be similar to the survival with an impaired PS due to extensive disease (Livingston and others, 1982). These data seem to indicate that PS only when it reflects the total body tumour load is a very strong prognostic factor. Objectively measurable parameters to replace the subjective estimation of PS would mean a big gain for the selection of patients for treatment and for the comparison of different studies. However, to our knowledge no relevant data are available to explain the biological basis for tumour-induced impairment of PS. Cohen and others (1981) have found that hemoglobin and albumin could be used as an alternative for PS. This finding is not supported by Osterlind and Andersen (1986), Souhami and others (1985), Cerny and others (1987) and Vincent and others (1987).

"NEW" PROGNOSTIC FACTORS

Recently three papers have been published and one is in press (Souhami and others, 1985; Osterlind and Andersen, 1986; Cerny and others, 1987; Vincent and others, 1987), in which by means of a multivariate analysis of a large number of pretreatment characteristics the value of laboratory parameters as an addition to or a replacement of the usual staging procedures has been investigated.

In table 1 the staging procedures, used in these 4 studies, are shown and compared with the staging procedures of the EORTC-study 08825 (Splinter and others, 1986). Osterlind and Andersen (1986) determined the extent of disease outside the thorax by bone marrow and liver investigation. Skeleton, retroperitoneal nodes and adrenals were not taken into consideration. Souhami and others (1985) performed a bone scan in all patients, only part of the patients underwent a bone marrow biopsy and investigation of the liver was performed only in the presence of abnormal liver function tests. They may have missed patients with extensive disease due to metastases in bone marrow, liver, adrenals and retroperitoneal nodes. Cerny and others (1987) investigated the bone marrow routinely, but looked for liver and bone metastases only if indicated by abnormal laboratory values. Retroperitoneal nodes and adrenals were not considered. It is important to realize that data from the EORTC-study 08825 indicate that 30% of patients with extensive disease and normal liver function tests (n = 81) had liver metastases, detected by ultrasound and/or CT-scanning. Vincent and others (1987)

Table 1   Comparison of staging procedures

	Osterlind 1	Souhami 2	Cerny 3	Vincent 4	EORTC 5
study n°					
phys. exam	+	+	+	+	+
perf. status	+	+	+	+	+
Hb-WBC-platelets	+	+	+	+	+
chemistry	+	+	+	+	+
chest X-ray	+	+	+	+	+
chest CT-scan	-	-	-	-	optional
abdomen CT-scan	-	-	-	-	+
or		if	if		and/or
abdomen ultrasound	-	indicated	indicated	+	+
bone scan	-	+	if indicated	+	+
brain CT-scan	if indicated	if indicated	if indicated	if indicated	if indicated
bone marrow	+	partly	+	+	+
bronchosc. + biopsy	+	+	+	+	+
peritoneoscopy	+	-	-	-	-
liver biopsy	+	-	-	-	-
n° of patients	778	371	407	333	681

investigated the liver, bone marrow and skeleton routinely. It is obvious that assignment of ` patients as having LD or ED in the 4 studies is not quite comparable. At the same time it should be recognized that no data are available about the relative importance of the site of metastases, detected by modern techniques such as second or third generation CT-scanners and ultrasound. In table 2 the independent prognostic variables in the 4 studies are shown.

Table 2   Comparison of independent prognostic variables

study n° 1 Osterlind	study n° 2 Souhami	study n° 3 Cerny	study n° 4 Vincent
PS	PS	PS	PS
extent	extent	extent	liver mts
LDH	alk. phosph.	LDH	alanine transaminase
hemoglobin	albumin	alk. phosph.	albumin
sodium		sodium	
(only in LD)	sodium	bicarbonate	
urate			
(only in LD)			

In all 4 studies PS remained an independent prognostic variable despite the different laboratory parameters, which contradicts the results of Cohen and others (1981). Furthermore in the first 3 studies extent of disease is an important independent prognostic variable, whereas in the study of Vincent and others (1987), who performed the most extensive staging, liver metastases remain an independent prognostic variable. However, in both study no 1, 2 and 4 the influence of stage of disease could be ignored without major loss of prognostic information. A conclusion about the relative value of the various laboratory parameters is hampered by the fact that not the same parameters were included in the different studies.

The authors of the first three studies conclude that by the addition of laboratory parameters to PS and extent of disease 3 - 5 different subgroups can be delineated. Vincent and others (1987) conclude that by using PS, albumin and alanine transaminase 3 prognostic subgroups can be delineated and they propose to replace the conventional staging system of LD and ED by their 3 parameters.

DATA FROM EORTC-STUDY 08825

From August 1982 till March 1986 681 patients were entered into the EORTC-study 08825, which investigated the role of maintenance chemotherapy. Patients were stratified at entry according to PS and extent of disease, treated with 5 courses of chemotherapy and randomized to follow up or 7 more courses if they had a major response or stable disease. This study design gives the possibility to investigate the importance of prognostic factors for survival from time of registration and from time of randomization. The following prognostic factors have been investigated: weight loss: < 1%, 1 - 5%, > 5%; age: < 50, 50 - 60, 60 - 70; sex; PS: ECOG 0 - 1 and 2 - 3; extent of disease: LD and ED; SGOT, SGPT, LDH, alkaline phosphatase: normal and abnormal. The laboratory parameters were used both separate and combined as a group.

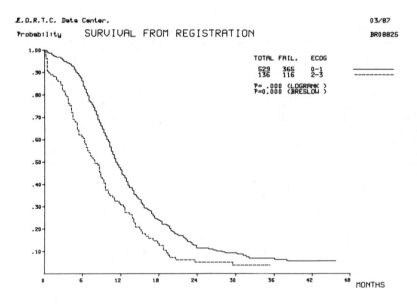

Fig. 1.   Survival of patients with PS-ECOG 0 + 1 and 2 + 3 from time of registration. The difference is highly significant.

In a univariate analysis all the prognostic factors except weight loss, age and sex were highly significantly correlated with survival from registration. PS and alkaline phosphatase were no longer significant (p < 0.08 Log Rank analysis) for survival from the time of randomization. The survival curves of the two PS-groups from registration and randomization (fig. 1 and 2) show that PS seems to be most important for the survival during the first month after start of treatment, which does not correspond with the conclusion of Ihde and others (1981) that even after a CR has been achieved PS still influenced survival. In table 3 the reasons are described why patients were not randomized after 5 courses of chemotherapy.

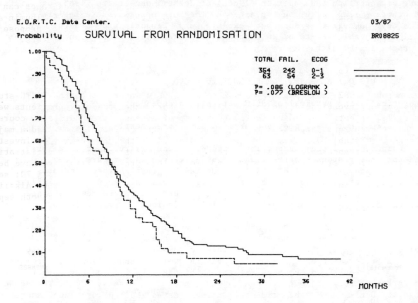

Fig. 2.   Survival of patients with PS-ECOG 0 + 1 and 2 + 3 from time of randomization. The difference is no longer significant.

Patients with progressive disease, treatment refusals, patients with excessive toxicity and early death were selected from the group, which did not reach randomization (table 3). In a cross table analysis we investigated which of the aforementioned prognostic factors by extent of disease were significantly different between the selected non-randomized patients and the randomized group.

Table 3   Reasons for leaving the study before randomization

Progression of disease	94	(43%)
Treatment refused	43	(20%)
Excessive toxicity	36	(16.5%)
Ineligible	13	
Early death	12	(58%)
Appearance of brain metastases	10	
Protocol violation	9	
Lost to follow up	3	
Other	11	

Only a performance status 2 + 3 in extensive disease patients was significantly different. This data suggest that a group of patients, which is at risk of early death after the first course of chemotherapy and should perhaps receive a different treatment, is mainly responsible for the difference in survival between the two PS-groups. A similar group of patients is presented by Morittu and others at this conference.

When a Cox multivariate analysis was performed it was found that only PS and extent of disease were independent prognostic factors for survival. Both separate and combined the liver function tests were not independent of extent of disease. This difference between the multivariate analysis of the EORTC study and the study of Osterlind and Andersen (1986a) of Souhami and others (1985) and of Cerny and others (1987) might be explained by the more extensive staging procedures in our study. However this does not explain why Vincent and others (1987) find alanine transaminase to be an independent prognostic factor, even independent of liverscanning by ultrasound.

BIOLOGICAL BASES FOR PROGNOSTIC FACTORS

Theoretically the survival of SCLC-patients is dependent of:

A.   The residual total body tumour load after treatment.

The residual total body tumour load depends on the pretreatment total body tumour load and the response to treatment. The latter two factors are strongly correlated (Ihde and others, 1981; Maurer and Pajak, 1981; Harper and others, 1982; Souhami and others, 1985) which is not very surprising since a 2 log cellkill in the presence of 10^{10} malignant cells will produce a complete remission and in the presence of 10^{11} malignant cells a partial remission. However this correlation is not absolute. Both in LD and ED patients non-responders exist and a small percentage of ED patients are longterm survivors.

Although methods become available to test the chemosensitivity of SCLC in vitro (Carney, this issue) it is not possible to predict the degree of response in vivo. Therefore major prognostic factors will be those, which are related to total body tumour load, such as extent of disease, PS, (Ihde and others, 1981) and intra thoracic tumour volume in LD (Harper and others, 1982). The negative prognostic influence of hepatic metastases, as described by Ihde and others (1981), may even not be related to the site of metastases but to the volume of the metastases, since the liver can harbour a lot of tumour. The majority of the other prognostic factors, listed in table 2 are probably somehow related to the total tumour volume, although this has not been proven and a possible relationship is not easy to understand. For example albumin, according to Vincent and others (1987) is correlated with the number of metastatic sites, with liver involvement and with hyponatremia. In the study of Souhami and others (1985) albumin is an independent prognostic factor next to sodium and surprisingly in the study of Cerny and others (1987) sodium is an independent prognostic factor, whereas albumin has no significant impact at all. Reasons for a lowered albumin level are pre-illness condition, decreased production, break down and dilution.

To our knowledge no data are available to understand the pathophysiology of hypoalbuminemia in SCLC or cancer in general. Therefore the above mentioned differences are difficult to explain. If a lowered albumin level is directly correlated to total tumour volume it is difficult to understand why it has no prognostic significance in the study of Cerny and others (1987). If however hypoalbuminemia is the resultant of a low pre-illness level due to e.g. alcohol abuse and dilution due to water retention, which may occur in a high percentage of patients (Comis and others, 1980), the importance of the albumin level may differ between patient populations and may indicate that some patients should be treated in a different way, because of hepatic insufficiency.

It is beyond doubt that the distinction in LD and ED is a very crude way to measure the total body tumour load. Therefore any additional laboratory parameter, which will give more detailed information about the tumour load, will have prognostic significance. However it is important to find out which of the avail-

able parameters give the best information and to understand why. Hopefully in the
near future a monoclonal antibody will be available to estimate the total body
tumour load.

B.   The growth rate of the residual tumour load after treatment.

Very few studies, all using an isotope labelling technique, have been performed
to measure the growth rate of lung cancer (Brigham, 1982). As recently published
(Splinter and others, 1987 a) we have performed serial measurements of neuron-
specific enolase (NSE) in SCLC-patients. Figure 3 shows a classical example of
the course of NSE during treatment. At the start of treatment an increased level
of NSE is found, which drops to a normal plateau between 5 and 10 ng/ml after the
first course of chemotherapy, if a major response is achieved. At the time of
progression an exponential rise of NSE occurs until death. From the exponential
rise of NSE the NSE doubling time (NSE-Td) can be calculated. The survival from

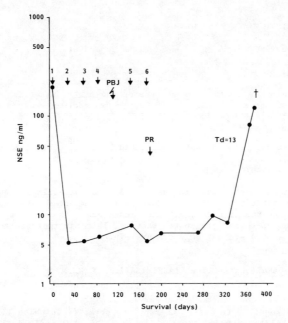

Fig. 3.   Serial NSE-measurements during treatment and follow up of SCLC is a
           patients, treated with 6 courses of chemotherapy.

the last normal NSE value till death is called survival from NSE rise. Of 31
patients enough data were availabe to calculate NSE-Td, which varied from 10 to
94 days. The spontaneous survival of these 31 patients from rise of NSE varied
from 1 to 11 months as shown in fig. 4! A linear regression curve showed a highly
significant correlation (p < 0.001) between the survival from NSE rise and NSE-
Td. If it is assumed that the exponential rise of NSE is an illustration of the
exponential growth of the tumour, it may be concluded that the survival from rise
of NSE is dependent of the tumour doubling time and the tumour load (Splinter and
others, 1987 b). The slope of the survival curve (fig. 4), is typical for the
group of intermediate survivors in SCLC, who are continuously at risk of dying.
These data support the theory that the growth rate of the residual tumour load
after treatment may be a prognostic factor independent of the degree of response.
It may explain why some complete responders survive relatively short and why some
partial responders survive relatively long.

No prognostic factors are known, which are correlated with the growth rate of SCLC. Perhaps pretreatment NSE-Td may provide some information.

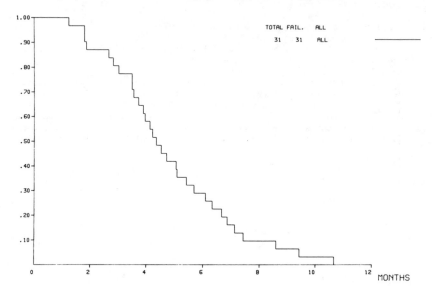

Fig. 4.   Survival from rise of NSE, unaffected by treatment, in 31 patients

C.   Pre-illness health?

Very little is known about the influence of the pre-illness general health condition of the patient on survival. However it seems reasonable to assume that the influence of the tumour on PS, albumin level etc. is also dependent of the pre-illness state of these prognostic factors. This may indicate that pretreatment prognostic factors are not only tumour-related.

THEORETICAL CONSIDERATIONS ABOUT A CLASSIFICATION OF SCLC.

Classification is required to select therapy, to stratify in phase III trials and to ensure comparability between studies. In case of the individual patient it will be most desirable to know whether he belongs to the group of early or intermediate death or to the group of longterm survivors.
By combining "old and new" prognostic factors subgroups with significantly different "good, intermediate and poor" survival curves can be obtained (fig. 5).
The main differences between the 3 curves occur in the first 1 - 3 months and after approx. 1 - 1.5 years, in between they run parallel and represent a population of patients, which is continuously at risk of dying. The slope of the curves suggests that basically the patient population can be divided into 3 groups: those who die early after the start of treatment, those who are alive at 1.5 - 2 years and those who die in between. However, these clinically very important 3 groups can not yet be distinguished by prognostic factors.
If the value of additional locoregional therapy, such as radiotherapy or surgery, is investigated, more extensive staging procedures than are recommended routinely (Ihde, 1985) will be needed to exclude as many ED-patients as possible.
Therefore the main use of a classification of SCLC, both the "old" and the "new" one will be to obtain comparable groups in randomized phase III trials and to allow comparison of patient groups in different studies all over the world.

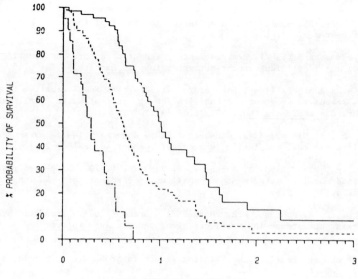

YEARS SINCE PRIMARY DIAGNOSIS

Fig. 5.   Three prognostic subgroups with a "good" "intermediate" and "poor" survival, based on PS, albumin and alanine transaminase.
From Vincent and others (1987)

Since laboratory measures are easily obtained objective parameters, not dependent
of the refinement of the tools or the skill of its user, such as the CT-scanner
and its radiologists, or of the experience of the clinician to estimate PS, it
should be investigated on an international scale whether the addition of laboratory parameters to PS and extent of disease or even replacement of the latter two
prognostic factors by laboratory parameters alone will produce a classification
of SCLC, which is equivalent or better than the existing one for the two purposes
mentioned above. If extent of disease will remain an important prognostic factor,
it will be essential to find out whether the site of metastases e.g. the liver or
the number of sites of metastases will give the most prognostic information.
These important data can not be learned from the 4 studies (Osterlind and Andersen, 1986; Souhami and others, 1985; Cerny and others, 1987; Vincent and others,
1987) because of the different staging procedures, which were used. Hopefully,
analysis of the EORTC-data may give an answer to this question, since extensive
staging data, laboratory parameters and the possibility to perform an analysis
from the time of randomization, including the response to treatment, are available as prognostic factors .
In 1988 the EORTC-Lung Cancer Group will organize a workshop on this difficult
and fascinating subject.

    ACKNOWLEDGEMENT

The members of the EORTC Lung Cancer Group are:
T. Splinter, J. McVie, O. Dalesio, A. Kirckpatrick, J. Burghouts, P. Postmus,
C. Veenhof, G. Giaccone, G. Kho, W. Bakker, G. ten Velde, C. Vendrik, N. van
Zandwijk, F. Palmen, K. Rozendaal, M. v.d. Burg, F. v. Breukelen,   M. Rinaldi,
J. Gracia, J. Kleisbauer, J. Wils, G. Miech, J. Festen, S. Wagenaar.

We are grateful to Amirpa van Eer for typing the manuscript.

REFERENCES

Brigham, B. (1982). Small cell anaplastic carcinoma of the lung. Cancer Chemo-
    ther. Pharmacol. 9, 1 - 5.

Cerny, T. and others (1987). Pretreatment prognostic factors and scoring system
    in 407 small-cell lung cancer patients. Int. J. Cancer 39, 146 -149.

Cohen, M. H. and others (1981) Laboratory parameters as an alternative to perfor-
    mance status in prognostic stratification of patients with small cell lung
    cancer. Cancer Treatm. Rep. 65, 187 - 195.

Comis, R. L., M. Miller, S. J. Ginsberg (1980). Abnormalities in water homeosta-
    sis in small cell anaplastic lung cancer. Cancer 45, 2414 - 2421.

Einhorn, L. H., W. H. Band, N. Hornback, J. Beng-Tek (1978). Long-term results in
    combined modality treatment of small cell carcinoma of the lung. Sem. in
    Oncol. 5, 309 - 313.

Giannone, L., D. H. Johnson, K.R. Hande, F. Greco (1987). Favorable prognosis
    of brain metastases in small cell lung cancer. Ann. Intern. Med. 106, 386-
    389.

Green, R. A and others (1969). Alkylating agents in bronchogenic carcinoma.
    Am. J. Med. 46, 516 - 525.

Harper, P. G. (1982). Tumor size, response rate, and prognosis in small cell
    carcinoma of the bronchus treated by combination chemotherapy. Cancer
    Treatm. Rep. 66, 463 - 470.

Hirsch, F. R., H. H. Hansen, B. Hainau (1979). Bilateral bone-marrow examinations
    in small cell anaplastic carcinoma of the lung. Acta Pathol. Microbiol.
    Scand. 87, 59 - 62.

Ihde, D. C. and others (1981). Prognostic implications of stage of disease and
    sites of metastases in patients with small cell carcinoma of the lung
    treated with intensive combination chemotherapy. Am. Rev. Respir. Dis. 123,
    500 - 507.

Ihde, D. C. (1985). Staging evaluation and prognostic factors in small cell lung
    cancer. In: Lung Cancer. Ed. J. Aisner. Churchill Livingstone New York. 241
    - 268.

Jacobs, H., M. J. Santicky, R. G. Stoller (1980). A comparison of survival in
    subjects of patients with extensive small cell lung carcinoma of the lung.
    Proc. Am. Soc. Clin. Oncol. 21, 455.

Livingston, R. B. and others (1982). Isolated pleural effusion in small cell lung
    carcinoma: favorable prognosis. A review of the Southwest Oncology Group
    experience. Chest 81, 208 - 211.

Maurer, L. H. and T.F. Pajak (1981). Prognostic factors in small cell carcinoma
    of the lung: a cancer and leukemia study. Cancer Treatm. Rep. 65, 767 - 774.

Mirra, P., J. E. Miziara, C. A. Schneider, B. Guida Filho (1982). Exploratory
    laparotomy in the detection of abdominal metastases of primary lung cancer.
    Int. Surg. 66, 141 - 143.

Orr, S. T. and J. Aisner (1986). Performance status assessment among oncology
    patients: a review. Cancer Treatm. Rep. 70, 1423 - 1429.

Osterlind, K. and P. K. Andersen (1986). Prognostic factor in small cell lung

cancer: Multivariate model based on 778 patients treated with chemotherapy
with or without irradiation. Cancer Res. 46, 4189 - 4194.

Pagani, J. J. (1983). Normal adrenal glands in small cell lung carcinoma: CT-
guided biopsy. A.J.R. 140, 949 - 951.

Smyth, J. F. and H. H. Hansen (1985). Current status of research into small cell
carcinoma of the lung: summary of the second workshop of the international
association for the study of lung cancer (IASLC). Eur. J. Clin. Oncol. 21,
1295 - 1298.

Splinter, T. A. W. and others (1986). EORTC 08825: induction versus induction
plus maintenance chemotherapy (CT) in small cell lung cancer. ASCO Proceedings 5, 188.

Splinter, T. A. W. and others (1987a). Neuron-specific enolase as a guide to the
treatment of small cell lung cancer. Eur. J. Cancer Clin. Oncol. 23, 171-
176.

Splinter, T. A. W. and others (1987b). Doubling time of neuron-specific enolase
and survival in small cell lung cancer patients. Results of a preliminary
analysis. Eur. J. Resp. Dis. Suppl. 149, 37 - 44.

Stahel, R., and others (1985). Detection of bone marrow metastasis in small cell
lung cancer by monoclonal antibody. J. Clin. Oncol. 3, 455 - 461.

Souhami, R. L. and others (1985). Prognostic significance of laboratory parameters measured at diagnosis in small cell carcinoma of the lung. Cancer Res.
45, 2878 - 2882.

Vincent, M. D., S. E. Ashley, I. E. Smith (1987). Prognostic factors in small
cell lung cancer: a simple prognostic is better than conventional staging.
In press in Eur. J. Cancer Clin. Oncol.

Zelen, M. (1973). Keynote address on biostatistics and data retrieval. Cancer
Chemother. Rep. 4, 31.

Diagnostic Imaging: Conventional Radiology, CT Scan and NMR: Alternative or Complementary?

R. Musumeci, L. Balzarini, J. D. Tesoro Tess,
R. Petrillo and E. Ceglia

Department of Diagnostic Radiology and Magnetic
Resonance, National Cancer Institute, Milano, Italy

ABSTRACT

Diagnostic radiology, including the newest MRI, has a very important place in the
diagnosis and staging of small cell lung carcinoma. The different investigations
have to be proposed in order to give an answer to the classical questions about
T, N and M. The diagnostic tools appear to be complementary and their major indications are discussed.

KEYWORDS

Small cell lung cancer; diagnostic imaging; conventional radiology; computerized
tomography; magnetic resonance imaging.

INTRODUCTION

Small cell lung cancer represents for the diagnostic radiologist as well as for
the radiotherapist and oncologist a great challenge both for diagnosis and staging. This particular lung cancer shows in fact a wide spectrum of presentations,
but the most important characteristic is represented by its typical attitude to
an early dissemination.
Obviously the diagnosis of this disease is clinical and histological but radiology plays a very important role in staging local disease and distant metastases.
Unlike bronchogenic carcinoma in fact oat cell cancer has prognosis and survival
less depending on mediastinal involvement than whether the disease has distant
metastases.
The staging system for primary lung cancer defined by the American Joint Committee, based on the TNM Classification is essentially oriented to predict surgical
resectability of the disease, thus failing to provide useful information for the
majority of patients with small cell carcinoma. The most widely applied staging
system is that of the Veterans Administration Lung Cancer Study Group.
This classification divides the patients in two distinct groups: patients with
limited disease (that could be encompassed in a single radiation field) or widespread disease. According to the literature (2) the most commonly involved organs are bone (19 - 38%), liver (18 - 34%), lymph nodes (16 - 55%), bone marrow
(11 - 47%), brain (0 - 14%), soft tissues (3 - 11%) and opposite lung (7 - 8%).
The ultimate diagnosis of small cell lung cancer is histologic, usually performed
by sputum cytology, needle aspiration, mediastinoscopy or thoracotomy, but the

first diagnostic approach in a patient with (or even without specific symptoms)
is currently performed by radiology. The diagnostic radiologist has the possibility to use a large series of diagnostic tools ranging from standard X-ray, to
CT and more recently to MRI (7).
And immediatly some questions arise:
- are all these procedures adequate?
- are them complementary or alternative?
- are them mandatory in each patient?
- which can be selected as the best algorithm?

CONVENTIONAL RADIOLOGY

The standard approach includes chest X-ray, always in double projection, better
if with high voltage. The primary tumor can usually go detected with this simple,
fast, widely available procedure in the great majority of the cases (1 - 10).
As regards hilar and/or mediastinal nodes, routine radiography can demonstrate
disease in a good percentage of patients, due to the characteristic bulk of the
nodes in this disease. This procedure usually also provides adequate assessment
of other sites of possible dissemination, such as contralateral lung, pleural or
pericardial effusions, involvement by contiguity or embolization of chest bones
(6 - 7 - 9).
Linear tomography can also improve the diagnosis of nodal involvement, both in
the standard orthogonal planes as well as in the 55° posterior oblique. Obviously the discovering of abnormal nodes appears to be strictly dependant on their
size (usually large in small cell carcinoma) and location. In fact nodes in the
hilar and paratracheal area can go easily detected while deep nodes, such as
subcarinal, can be missed even with radiographs of good quality (4 - 5 - 6 - 9).

COMPUTERIZED TOMOGRAPHY

Dynamic CT usually gives a much better picture of the extent of disease than routine radiography and linear tomography in lung cancer (1 - 3 - 4 - 5 - 6 - 9):
this is also true in small cell carcinoma patients. With a state of the art CT
(including the use of the newest machines, injection of contrast medium for angio
CT, carefull positioning of the patient and adequate slice covering of the whole
chest), more nodal areas as well as more non nodal disease such as lung nodules,
effusions (pleural or pericardial), bone changes and soft tissue swellings can
be detected.
The statistical evaluation of the diagnostic possibilities of the different radio
logical procedures are reported in Table 1, according to Glazer (6) in a group of
patients with lung carcinoma, including 10 cases of oat cell disease.
Reported data and personal experience suggest that CT gives a much better picture
of the extent of disease than routine radiography in oat cell carcinoma patients.
More nodal areas are seen with CT than routine radiography. However, routine radiography on the initial pretherapy examinations demonstrates that mediastinal or
hilar involvement was noted in almost all cases with small cell carcinoma and pathology present. More non nodal disease was seen on the pretherapy CT examinations but, if the mediastinal area is noted to have metastatic disease by routine
radiography, is this added information necessary to provide rational treatment?
It is difficult to advocate the routine use of chest CT in oat cell carcinoma patients when enough staging information can be obtained from routine chest radiography. The role of CT in these patients is probably more significant in the evaluation for distant sites of metastase.

TABLE 1   Evaluation of different radiological procedures in
           staging hilar and mediastinal nodes in lung cancer
           (Glazer 1983)

* Procedure	RX		Tomogr.		CT	
* n° cases	120		79		120	
+/+	54	(45%)	52	(65.8%)	83	(69.2%)
+/-	12	(10%)	7	(8.9%)	4	(3.3%)
-/+	31	(25.8%)	9	(11.4%)	3	(2.5%)
-/-	23	(19.2%)	11	(13.9%)	30	(25%)
Sensitivity	54/85 = 63.5%		52/61 = 85.2%		83/86 = 96.2%	
Specificity	23/35 = 65.7%		11/18 = 61.1%		30/34 = 88.2%	
Accuracy	77/120 = 64.2%		63/79 = 79%		113/120 = 94.1%	

===

MAGNETIC RESONANCE IMAGING

More recently MRI has been included among the diagnostic tools in staging a
number of different neoplasms. The experience with this new imaging modality is,
almost in our country, still initial (10) but the results appear to be highly
suggestive.
This new non radiological imaging technique has the unique possibility to acquire images in every spatial plane with the same quality (multiplanarity). The si-
gnal that emerges from the different body tissues represents the actual status
of these tissues (i.e. chemical composition, water content, proton density, proton relaxation times, ect.). With this technique it is possible to acquire images representative of all the different components of tissue's signals (multi-
parametricity). Further, imaging the chest, the mandatory need of ECG gating during acquisition produces sharp, clear, frozen images of the chest and its content. The high contrast latitude of MRI allows a wide spectrum of information
about chest walls, pleura, lung parenchima, mediastinum, vessels, pericardium,
hearth and bones.
Our personal experience with this new diagnostic procedure is still in progress,
but some considerations can be drawn. For lesions of the lung parenchima, CT can
be considered the investigation of choice, due to its very high image resolu-
tion. The same considerations are of value for the demonstration of small pleural implants, initial invasion of the chest walls or ribs destruction. The hila
and the mediastinum on the contrary appear to be anatomical regions where MRI is
adequate for diagnosis.
As regards the problem of staging metastatic nodes (N1 and N2) in lung cancer,
the first results of MRI compared with histologic findings are reported in Table
2.
The diagnostic results of MRI can be compared with those obtained with CT. This
technique in fact is usually considered as the most accurate procedure for staging mediastinal nodes (N2) in lung cancer (3 - 4 - 5 - 6 - 9). The results of
the comparison are reported in Table 3. As clearly appears from this table, the
statistical results of CT and MRI in staging mediastinal nodes in lung cancer
are very similar. MRI has in our hands higher sensitivity and percentage of pre-
dictivity of a negative report while CT demonstrated higher specificity and pre-

dictivity of positive reports. The values of overall diagnostic accuracy are on
the contrary statistically the same (84.3% v.s. 85.7%).

TABLE 2   Comparison MR/Hist. in the evaluation of N_2 para-
           meter in 28 patients with lung cancer

	MR/HIST		
+/+	+/-	-/-	-/-
10	3	1	14

Accuracy = 24/28   (85.7%)

TABLE 3   Comparison MR/CT in patient with lung cancer

	Sensitivity %	Specificity %	Predictive + value %	Predictive - value %	Accuracy %
CT	79	89	82.3	84.4	84.3
MR	90.2	82.4	76.9	93.3	85.7

SUMMARY OF THE PROCEDURES FOR T AND N

In conclusion we can consider that standard X-ray, with or without linear tomography, appears to be generically adequate for the diagnosis of small cell cancer of the lung and for staging its loco-regional diffusion. These simple procedures are mandatory in each diagnostic and therapeutic protocol for the disease.
Computerized radiology (CT and MRI) usually improves the accuracy mainly for staging nodes, but this contribution is not always accepted as necessary for treatment.
Anyway if we want to supply our patients with an exhaustive diagnostic staging
of their thoracic disease before treatment, conventional radiology, CT and MRI
must be considered as complementary.

EVALUATION OF M

The staging of M parameter (i.e. distant metastases) can be summarized as follows:
1) Isotopic bone scan is enough accurate for excluding bone metastases: this in-
    vestigation, when abnormal, has to be completed with conventional X-ray ske-
    letal survey.
2) MRI is at now considered as the single most sensitive imaging modality for
    brain disease and for this reason it must be applied as the investigation of
    choice, eventually alternated with contrast CT.
3) Ultrasounds are adequate to assess liver and adrenals in a fast, cheap, easy
    repeatable way and this must be the first diagnostic step. Contrast CT with
    fast bolus injection can be considered the investigation of choice. The expe-
    rience with MRI in this area is at the beginning and needs further studies:
    with the most up to date scan software programs (fast scan) the results ap-
    pear promising.

REFERENCES

Bragg D.G., Rubin P. and Youker J.E. (1985) Oncologic imaging. Pergamon Press, New York.

Clavel M., Rebattu P. and Trillet V. (1987) The clinical importance of a well designed clinical, biochemical and instrumental follow up program. International Conference on Small Cell Lung Cancer, Ravenna - March 27-28, Abstract Book, 57-62.

Frederick H.M., Bernardino M.E., Baron M., Colvin R., Mansour K and Miller J. (1984) Accuracy of chest computerized tomography in detecting malignant hilar and mediastinal involvement by squamous cell carcinoma of the lung. Cancer 54, 2390-2395.

Glazer G.M., Francis I.R., Shirazi K.K., Bookstein F.L., Gross B.H. and Orringer M.B. (1983) Evaluation of the pulmonary hilum: comparison of conventional radiography, 55° posterior oblique tomography and dynamic computed tomography. J. Comp. Ass. Tomogr. 7, 983-989.

Khan A., Gersten K.C., Carvey J., Khan F.A. and Steinberg H. (1985) Oblique hilar tomography, computed tomography and mediastinoscopy for prethoracotomy staging of bronchogenic carcinoma. Radiology 156, 295-298.

Lewis E., Bernardino M.E., Valdivieso M., Farha P., Barnes P. and Thomas J.L. (1982) Computed tomography and routine chest radiography in oat cell carcinoma of the lung. J. Comp. Ass. Tomogr. 6, 739-745.

Musumeci R. (1987) Principi di radiodiagnostica oncologica. Manuale di Oncologia medica, Masson Italia Editori, 63-106.

Musumeci R., Balzarini L., Ceglia E., Petrillo R., Tesoro Tess J.D., Preda F., Ravasi G., Pastorino U. and Valente M. (1986) MRI of mediastinal lymph node metastases (N2) in patients with primary lung cancer: perspective study. SMRM - Fifth Annual Meeting, Montreal 19-22 Agosto.

Osborne D.R., Korobkin M., Ravin C.E., Putman C.E., Wolfe W.G., Sealy W.C., Young W.G., Breiman R., Heaston D., Ram P. and Halber M. (1982) Comparison of plain radiography, conventional tomography and computed tomography in detecting intrathoracic lymph node metastases from lung carcinoma. Radiology 142, 157-161.

Steckel R.J. and Kagan A.R. (1976) Diagnosis and staging of cancer. A radiological approach. W.B. Saunders Co, Philadelphia.

Fiberoptic Bronchoscopy in the Diagnosis and Control of the Evolution of Small Cell Anaplastic Carcinoma

L. Spiga, M. Patelli, V. Poletti and
M. Simonetti

Servizio di Broncologia e Fisiopatologia Respiratoria,
Ospedale Bellaria, Bologna, Italy

ABSTRACT

The Authors present their experience on bronchoscpic approach to the diagnosis
of small cell lung cancer.

KEYWORDS

Small cell lung cancer; fiberoptic bronchoscopy.

Lung cancer originating in the cells of bronchial mucosa has a predictable dis
semination pattern which depends on lung anatomy. Dissemination occurs along the
lymphatic vessels that run through the peribronchovascular region and the inter
lobular septa, the axial and peripheral connective tissue and, more rarely, on
the surface of the respiratory spaces. Spencer [1] identified two large groups
of bronchogenic carcinomas, depending on their site of origin: central and peri
pheral lesions. The former originate in the bronchi that are macroscopiccally vi
sible, while the latter are observed in the bronchi that cannot be seen with a
naked eye. Heithzman [2], considering these anatomic classification, purposed
the following anatomic and radiological classification of bronchogenic carcinoma

        I - Central Lesions:
            A) Endobronchial growth
                1) Collapse
                2) Obstructive pneumonia
            B) Transbronchial growth
                1. Hilar mass
                2. Centrifugal extension
                    a) along the axial connective tissue
                    b) in the peribronchovascular lymphatics.
        II - Peripheral Masses:growth of "hilic" and of "lepidic" type
            A) Peripheral mass without obstruction of the centripetal
               lymph flow.
            B) Peripheral mass with obstruction of the centripetal

lymph flow in the hilar lymph nodes
C) Peripheral mass with obstruction of the lymph flow
   within the mass itself.

Fiberoptic bronchoscopy approach is different in according to the anatomic and
X-ray pictures of the condition. The central lesions with an endobronchial
growth pattern are easily identified by bronchial biopsies.At endoscopy central
lesions with transbronchial growth may show either infiltration or indirect
signs, such as extrinsic compression, hyperemia, rigidity or negative results.
If there is a hilar mass with a centrifugal extension, transbronchial pulmonary
biopsies can also be carried out in the involved region.

TABLE 1 Fiberoptic bronchoscopy approach to
bronchogenic carcinoma

Central Lesions	Endoscopy	Procedure
1) Endobronchial growth	- Positive	- Bronchial biopsy - Broncholavage
2) Transbronchial growth	- Positive - Indirect signs - Negative	
A) Hilar Mass		- Bronchial biopsy - Transbronchial needle aspiration - broncholavage
B) Hilar Mass with centrifugal extension		- Bronchial biopsy - Transbronchial needle aspiration - Transbronchial biopsy - broncholavage

In peripheral localized lesions the endoscopic pattern is normally negative and
targeted biopsies are performed under fluoroscopic control in all cases.

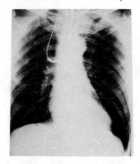

Fig. 1. Targeted biopsy of a right uppur lobe lesion
unser fluoroscopic control.

When there is a peripheral mass with obstruction of the centripetal limph-flow at the hilar level the endoscopic pattern may be negative or caracterized by indirect signs. In all these cases bronchial biopsies and transbronchial needle aspiration are performed in association with targeted biopsies.

TABLE 2 Fiberoptic bronchoscopy approach
to bronchogenic carcinoma

Peripheral lesions	Endoscopy pattern	Fiberoptic procedures
A) Peripheral mass without obstruction of the centripetal lymph-flow	Negative	- Targeted biopsy under Rx.control - TB Needle aspirat under Rx.control - Broncholavage
B) Peripheral mass with obstruction of the centripetal lymph flow in the hilar limph nodes	Negative Indirect signs	- Bronchial biopsy - Targeted biopsy - TB Needle Aspira tion - Broncholavage
C) Peripheral mass with obstruction of the limph-flow within the mass itself	Negative	- Targeted biopsy - TB Needle aspirat under Rx.control - Broncholavage

In neoplastic diffuse lung involvment

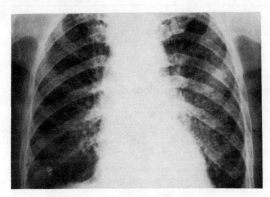

Fig. 2 Reticular Rx. pattern more evident on the left
lung representing a diffuse neoplastic lymphan
gitic spread.

the endoscopic pattern may be rarely positive and the fiberoptic procedures useful for the diagnosis are the transbronchial l ung biopsies and the bronchoalveolar lavage.

TABLE 3 Fiberoptic bronchoscopy approach
to bronchogenic carcinoma

Diffuse lung involvment	Endoscopic pattern	Fiberoptic procedures

A) Carcinomatous
   limphangitis
	Positive
	Indirect signs
	
	Negative
		- Bronchial biopsy
		- Transbronchial
		  lung biopsy
		- Alveolar lavage

B) Bronchiolo-alveolar carcinoma.		

Small cell anaplastic carcinoma is a type of bronchogenic carcinoma which has peculiar clinical, biological and genetic characteristics [3].
Our experience concerns 549 cases of small cell anaplastic carcinoma alla diagnosed with biopsy (520 bronchial biopsies and 29 transbronchial pulmonary biopsies). This histological pattern was found in 14.5% of the 3.776 primary malignant lung cancers diagnosed in our Centre. There was a prevalence of males(88%) over females - mean age was 62 years. X-ray were characterized by the following morphological aspects.

TABLE 4   Small cell anaplastic carcinoma - X-ray patterns
(Personal experience)

	N° Cases	%
Central lesions	470	86
. Collapse or obstructive pneumonia	302	55
. Hilar mass	168	31
Peripheral masses	74	13
. Coin lesions	24	4
. Coin masses with hilar involvment	50	9
Diffuse involvment	2	0.5
Negative	3	0.5
Pleural effusion	20	3

1) 470 central lesion (86%), 168 (31%) of which hilar masses and 302 (55%) with atelectasia and obstructive pneumonia.
2) 74 peripheral lesions (13%), 24 (4%) of which were coin lesions and 50 (9%)were peripheral masses with hilar involvment.
3) Diffused reticular lesions (0.5%). In 3 cases (0.5%), the X-rays did not show any pathological alterations. In 20 cases (3%) there was also a homolateral pleural effusion.

Endoscopy was characterized:

TABLE 5   Small cell anaplastic carcinoma. Endoscopic patterns
(Personal experience)

	N° CASES	%
. Concentric stenosis mucosal and/or submucosal infiltration	262	48
. Vegetation lesions	161	29
. Extrensic compression and mucosal infiltration	88	16
. Extrensic compression	14	2.5
. Negative	24	4.5

- Concentric stenosis due to mucosal and/or submucosal infiltration in 262 cases
  (48%);
- Vegetating in 161 cases (29%);
- Extrinsic compression and mucosal infiltration in 88 cases (16%)
- Extrinsic compression, rigidity and hyperemia in 14 cases (2.5%)
- Endoscopy was normal in 24 cases (4.5%).

The cytological investigation either with bronchial or bronchiolo-alveolar lavage was positive in 316 cases (58%), suspicious in 87 (15%) and negative in 146 cases (27%).

TABLE 6   Small cell anaplastic carcinoma. Diagnostic yield of
cytologic investigations
(Personal experience)

	N° CASES	%
. Negative (Class I-II)	146	27
. Suspicious (Class III)	87	15
. Positive (Class IV-V)	316	58

The diagnostic yield of bronchial biopsy in the lesions endoscopically visible is pratically 100%. In the central lesions characterized by a transbronchial growth pattern, the diagnostic yield ranges from 92 to 97%, using either bronchial biopsy and transbronchial needle aspiration [4]. In the peripheral masses, the transbronchial biopsies performed under X-ray control show size-related differences in diagnostic yield. In the lesions that have a diametre of less than 2 cm, the yield is 51%, whereas in those with a diametre between 2 and 6 cm, it is 78% [5]. In the radiologically diffused lesions that are the expression of carcinomatous lymphangitis, transbronchial biopsy may be diagnostic in 90% of cases [6]. The high sensitivity is becaouse transbronchial biopsy samples the centrilobular zone

and the structures of these zones are primary and diffusely involved in neopla
stic lymphangitic spread.
Transbronchial thin-needle biopsy is used for the diagnosis of central lesions
with transbronchial involvement, which are negative at endoscopy or show indi
rect signs, as well as to diagnose peripheral lesions. By using this technique,
a cytological investigation can be conducted which has a specificity - in terms
of hystotype identification - in less than 70% of cases, in our experience.
This metod is also used for bronchogenic carcinoma staging, by sampling the pa
ratracheal and peribronchial lymph nodes [7]. These staging procedures however,
are not important in small cell anaplastic carcinoma, since in this type of can
cer it is important to identify only a limited stage - involving the controlate
ral and mediastinic hilar lymph nodes - and an extended stage. Fiberoptic bron
choscopy is also used to control the evolution of the disease. Of the 30 cases
that were referred to our Centre for a long-term control at 3 to 36 months(mean
7 months), 27 cases were observed to show a regression of endoscopic and histo
pathological conditions. Finally, fiberoptic broncoscopy has recently become a
therapeutic instrument if combined to laser technology.
The YAG laser is useful in endobronchial obstructing neoplasms in which a surgi
cal approach is not indicated. Small cell carcinoma of the lung presents more
frequently as a central vegetating lesion and, in our experience, a laser treat
ment may be useful also before radio-chemiotherapy. In fact the ricanalization
of the bronchial tree may immediately improve the patient status.

REFERENCES

1. Spencer H. (1977). Pathology of the lung. Pergamon Press.

2. Heithzman E.R. (1984). The lung. Radiologic-Pathologic correlations.
   Mosby Co.

3. Fannuzzi M.G., Scoggin C.H. (1986). Small Cell Lung Cancer: State of Art.
   Am.Rev.Resp.Dis, 134: 593-608.

4. Shure D., Fevullo P.F. (1985). Transbronchial needle aspiration in the
   diagnosis of submucosal and peribronchial bronchogenic carcinoma. Chest,88:
   49-51.

5. Spiga L., Patelli M., Simonetti M., Zannoni D., Poletti V. (1985). Bronchial
   alveolar carcinoma: diagnostic usefulness of transbronchial lung biopsy.
   Rec.Prog.Med., 76: 459-464.

6. Poletti V., Patelli M., Simonetti M., Spiga L. et al. (1986). Carcinomatous
   lymphangitis of the lung. National Congress of Oncology, Monduzzi Ed.,
   1071-1078.

7. Wang K.P., Brower R., et al.: "Flexible Transbronchial Needle Aspiration for
   Staging of Bronchogenic Carcinoma. Chest, 84: 571-576 (1983).

Nuclear Medicine in Staging of Lung Cancer: Immunoscan in Detecting Small Metastatic Deposits

P. Riva

Nuclear Medicine Department, "M. Bufalini" Hospital
and Istituto Oncologico Romagnolo, Cesena, Italy

ABSTRACT

Immunoscintigraphy by means of antiCEA MoAb(FO23C5,Sorin Biomedica, Italy) labelled with ^{131}I or ^{111}In was carried out in a group of 111 patients bearing lung carcinomas.12 patients were affected with oat cell carcinoma;99 patients presented not small cell tumour.83 pa = tients were studied before surgery,while in 28 the radioimmuno= detection was performed after the operation.The results indicate the high diagnostic sensitivity achievable with this technique in the detection of primary tumours(80/83) as well as their associated lesions.The immunoscintigraphy led to the diagnosis of lymph node (17/19),brain(6/6),bone(27/34) and chest(3/3) metastases,allowing , in some cases, the detection of occult lesions.The outcomes were more favourable when the ^{111}In label was employed rather than ^{131}I compound.The results were more satisfactory in the group of not small cell carcinoma patients.Moreover, the employ of immuno- scintigraphy in those patients already submitted to operation may overcome the limits of radiological investigations wich are unable to differentiate fibrotic from neoplastic lesions.In 28 patients The lesions of the chest(9/10), of the lymph nodes(1/2), of the brain(3/3) and of the bones(19/22) were satisfactory identified.In this group 6 occult lesions later confirmed were shown.Finally 3 therapeutical applications were carried out in patients with advanced disease.In 2 patients i.v. treated,the clinical effect was very poor.In 1 patient with pleural neoplastic effusion the anti- bodies were intrapleurally repeatedely administered obtaining a reduction of pleural fluid and a complete disappearance of its neoplastic cells.

KEYWORDS

Lung cancer, radiolabelled monoclonal antibodies ,radioimmuno = detection,radioimmunotheraphy.

INTRODUCTION

The present availability of monoclonal antibodies raised against
tumour associated antigens for "in vivo" applications leads to an
innovative approach for the management of neoplastic patients. The
monoclonal antibodies are labelled with gamma rays emitting isoto-
pes enabling the external detection of the tumours. The same la =
belling procedure is carried out utilizing beta or alpha emitters
radioisotopes in order to concentrate on the neoplastic tissue a
high radiation dose aiming to destroy the malignancies. This "immunologic" approach presents many advantages:
-the specific detection of neoplastic tissue that is recognized by
means of an immunological reaction between the antigen expressed by
the tumour and the exogenous antibody. Thus the radioimmunodetection
give us specific informations concerning the kind of the investiga
ted lesions, whereas other methods (US,CT scan,NMR) can identify
the tumour on the basis of its morphological or topographical
changes;
-the immunoscintigraphy allows a whole study of the patients em =
ploying only one dose of radiolabelled MoAb. A complete staging of
the patient can be so achieved;
-in many cases the radioimmunodetection leads to the diagnosis of
occult lesions non detectable by means of other investigations:thus
more precocious   treatments can be applied. On the other hand the
employment,in humans, of exogenous murine MoAbs may cause early or
late immunologic side effects. These adverse reactions however are
uncommon,are dose depending and are further reduced by the use of
$F(ab')$ or $F(ab')_2$ fragments. The production of antimouse antibodies
in patients submitted to administration of a large amount(more
than 10 mg) of MoAbs , for therapeutical purposes ,is very frequent. The HAMA ,if a second or a third treatment is performed,
change the biodistribution of antitumour murine antibodies,decrease
their uptake in the cancer and shorten their effective half life.In
spite of the present limitations encountered in clinical applica =
tions of radiolabelled monoclonal antibodies, their usefulness for
the staging and follow up of neoplastic patients has been extensively investigated and many therapeutical clinical trials are in
progress. At present the tumours most studied by means of this new
technique are those from gastrointestinal tract,skin (melanoma)
and female genitalia while few studies have been reported on lung
cancers. On the basis of positive findings obtained in a wide im-
munohystochemical and serological study we decided to carry out the
radioimmunodetection in patients with different kind of lung cancer
and in 3 patients a therapeutical approach was tried.

MATERIALS

CEA Serology

Serum levels of CEA were determined by radioimmunoassay(CEA M-K ,
Sorin Biomedica,Italy) using a cut off value of 5 ng/ml.

Immunohystochemistry

The indirect immunoperoxidase studies(Garrigus and others,1982 ;
Sternberg,1979) were obtained in surgical or bioptical specimens
using the IMUCOLOR KIT (Sorin Biomedica,Italy).The neoplastic tissues were tested with two antibodies:F023C5(Sorin,Italy) and MoV
15(INT,Milan,Italy).Peroxidase activity was put in evidence using
3-amino-9-ethylcarbazole solution (20 mcg/ml) in 0,1 M Sodium ace-
tate,pH 4,9,containing 5% of M-Dimethylformamide and 0,02% Hydrogen
peroxide.

Monoclonal Antibodies

The antiCEA MoAb F023C5 recognize an epitope on the protein portion
of CEA and does not react with granulocytes(Buraggi,1984;Mariani ,
1984). Monoclonal immunoglobulins were purified from mouse ascitic
fluids by caprilic acid preparation and $F(ab')_2$ fragments were ge
nerated by pepsin digestion. Coupling of Diethylentriaminepentaacetic
acid (DTPA) to bivalent fragments was carried out using the bicy =
clic anhydride method (Hnatowich,Layne, Childs,1982). The $F(ab')_2$
DTPA fragments were radiolabelled by addition of 50-300 ml(74-111
MBq,i.e. 2-3 mCi) of sterile and pyrogen-free radioactive Indium
chloride (Amersham,England). More than 95% of the ^{111}In was bound
to the antibody as demonstrated by HPLC. The antiCEA $F(ab')_2$
fragments were labelled with ^{131}I too,using the iodogen method.
The immunoreactivity of both reagents was determined by means of
a direct binding assay(Wahl,Parker,Philpopt,1983). An ELISA method
was employed in order to determine both the development and the
serum title of human anti murine antibodies (HAMA) before and
after the administration of labelled MoAbs.

Immunoscintigraphy Protocol

When the ^{131}I labelled MoAb was used, the patients admitted to radioimmunodetection were treated by administering 30 drops (per day)
of Lugol's 2% solution starting 4 days before the injection and
continuing 5 days thereafter(Chatal, 1984). The use of ^{111}In radio
pharmaceutical avoids this procedure(Epenetos and others,1985). All
patients were submitted to skin test in both arms by injecting
3.0 mcg of antibodies intradermally. Routine clinical analyses to
evaluate the hematopoietic,hepatic and renal function were performed before the test and during the subsequent two weeks. The ra=
diolabelled antibody solution (5 ml) containing 111-185 MBq (3-5
mCi) of ^{111}In (Indomab-2 ,Sorin)or ^{131}I (Iodomab,Sorin) was inje=
cted intravenously over a 2 min period. Body distribution of mono
clonal antibodies was studied immediately after injection and at
multiple time intervals up to 120 hr by analogical and computerized scintigraphy. The optimal time for tumour imaging was found
to be between 48 and 72 hr for ^{111}In whereas resulted to be be=
tween 72 and 120 hr for ^{131}I radiopharmaceutical. Moreover when
^{131}I compound was used the dual tracer subtraction technique was
employed by injecting, prior of the immunoscan, 74 MBq (2 mCi) of
^{99m}Tc HSA or ^{99m}Tc colloid. In this case were recorded first the

^{131}I antibody image and immediately afterward ,the blood pool and
liver parenchima ^{99m}Tc images. In all patients whole body scans
were obtained with a large field of view gamma camera (LFOW,SIEMENS)
connected with   Eurobit System IDRA 80 computer for data proces-
sing. The patients were selected for immunoscintigraphy studies on
the basis both of CEA raised serum levels and/or of positive out -
comes obtained by means of immunostaining carried out employing the
FO23C5 MoAb on surgical or bioptical specimens.

Radioimmunotheraphy Protocol

3 patients bearing an epidermoid lung cancer in advanced stage of
disease, following failure of surgical,chemotheraphy and radiotherapy regimens, were submitted to a treatment with ^{131}I radiolabelled
MoAbs. The antibodies employed were in one case the antiCEA 494/32
(Bheringwerke,FRG) and in the remaining 2 patients the aforementioned FO23C5 The doses of immunoglobulins ranged between 5 and 20 mg,
the doses of ^{131}I ranged between 740 and 3700 MBq(20-100 mCi). In
2 cases the radiopharmaceutical was intravenously administered while
in 1 patient with an intractable pleural malignant effusion multiple (7) intrapleural injections(Hammersmith Oncology Group,1984 ;
Humm ,1986) were carried out.

RESULTS

Immunoperoxidase Studies

The in vitro studies of antigenic characteristics of neoplastic tis
sue have shown that most of the epitelial tumours are CEA expres -
sing. By contrast the small cell carcinomas do not produce this an
tigen but can be recognized by means of the MoAb MoV15. In this
group of cancers, however, CEA expressing cells,with methaplastic
changes, could be demonstrated on the tissue around the neoplastic
area. This my explain the positive outcomes obtained by means of in
vivo radioimmunodetection in the small cell carcinoma group (see
Table 1).

TABLE 1   Immunostaining of Lung Cancer

Antibody	Small Cell Ca.		Not Small Cell Ca	
	+	−	+	−
FO23C5	1	34	43	6
MoV15	23	4	34	0

Specimens studied n. 145

Immunoscintigraphy Studies

Primary tumours. 111 patients,99 bearing not small cell cancer and
12 bearing oat cell carcinoma, were submitted to radioimmunode =
tection. 83 were studied before surgical treatment while 28 were
investigated 3-12 months after the operation. The primary tumours
were detected in most of the cases,best results being achieved by
the use of ^{111}In compound (see Table 2).

TABLE 2 Immunoscintigraphy of Primary Lung Cancer

	^{131}I+	^{111}In+	TOTAL +
Small Cell Cancer	2 / 3	8 / 8	10/11(90,9%)
Not Small Cell Cancer	19/20	51/52	70/72(97,2%)

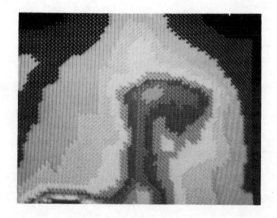

Fig.1. Immunoscintigraphic image of a epi=
dermoid cancer of left lung. The study was
performed 72 hr after the administration of
148 MBq of ^{111}In F(ab')$_2$ antiCEA. A strong
uptake in the tumour is clearly shown.
Note a quite non specific uptake in sternal
bone marrow. The background activity is
low.

The immunoscintigraphy approach to the study of primary lung tu=
mours was carried out with many purposes:
-The assesment of the method by administering the radiopharmaceu=
tical before the operation and by counting later the surgically re
sected specimens. Employing this technique we observed a signifi =
cant higher uptake in the tumour than in the normal parenchima get
ting a tumour to background ratio value of 5.
-The differential diagnosis of periferic lesions when bronchosco
py is negative and needle biopsy cannot be performed.
-The patient staging before operation. This particular application
in our experience, looks very promising. We succeeded in detecting
the primary tumour and at the same time , many associated local or
distant lesions (see Table 3 and Table 4).

Table 3 Immuno-cintigraphy of Primary Small Cell Lung Cancer
Associated Lesion Detected

Organs	$^{131}I+$	$^{111}In+$	TOTAL +
Bone	0/2	2/2	2./4
Nodes	–	2/2	2/2
Brain	–	1/1	1/1
Chest	3/3	–	3/3
			8/10 (80%)

Patients Studied n. 12

Table 4 Primary Not Small Cell Cancer
Associated Lesion Detected

Organs	$^{131}I+$	$^{111}In+$	TOTAL+
Bone	11/14	14/16	25/30
Nodes	5/5	10/12	15/17
Brain	2/2	3/3	5/5
Chest	1/1	2/2	3/3
ABDOMEN	1/1	1/1	2/2
			50/57(87,7%)

Patients Studied n. 71

We could image,in fact , mediastinal involved lymph nodes,neopla
stic spreading in the lung parenchima surrounding the tumour as
well as bone,brain and abdominal metastases (see Fig. 2 and Fig.3)

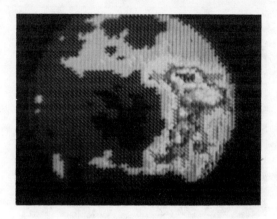

Fig.2 Epidermoid cancer of the upper left
lobe ,well imaged in subtracted image obtai
ned 72 hr after injection of 185 MBq^{131} I
antiCEA. At the same time a neoplastic sprea
ding in lower lobe,undetected by chest X ray,
is evident (anterior wiew).

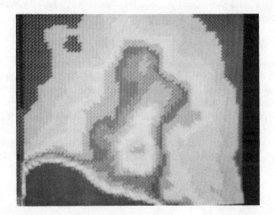

Fig.3 Small cell cancer of left hylar re =
gion. The uptake of ^{111}In antiCEA(MBq 148)
in the tumour is very high.Two metastatic
lymph nodes,in the upper mediastinum and in
right lower hylar region are detected too.

In some cases the immunoscintigraphy led to the detection of occult
metastases ,when other investigations resulted negative. These lesions were confirmed as true positive 6-8 months later by sub -
sequent follow up (see Fig. 4).

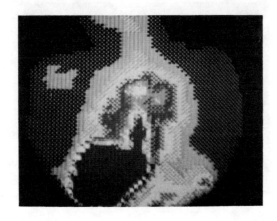

Fig. 4 Epidermoid left lung cancer clearly
imaged ,in anterior wiew 48 hr after inje =
ction of ^{111}In labelled F(ab')$_2$. Beside
the tumour two hot spots were found:in right
hylar region and in right shoulder correspon
ding respectively to unexpected lymph node
and bone metastases. These lesions were de =
tected by radiological investigations only
8 months later.

   Altogether the outcomes obtained demonstrate the usefulness of radioimmunodetection in imaging both not small cell and oat cell car
cinoma. Moreover the comparison between the ^{131}I and 111In radio =
pharmaceutical have put in evidence that this latter compound give better definite positive scan and lead to higher tumour to back
ground ratio, improving the sensitivity of the method. The positive
detection of small cell carcinomas,achieved in high percentage of
cases , is due to MoAbs' uptake in metaplastic areas surrounding
the tumour ,as shown in immunohistochemical studies. In some cases
the immunoscintigraphy resulted positive even if the chest X-ray ga
ve negative or doubtful outcomes. No positive images were observed
when using, as a negative control, an irrelevant antibody anti
HMWMAA (High Molecular Weight Melanoma Associated Antigen : MoAb
225.28S, Sorin ,Italy), radiolabelled with ^{99m}Tc.
Already operated patients   The radioimmunodetection was carried
out in 28 not small cell cancer patients already submitted to complete surgical removal of the tumour. In this group of patients is
necessary to differentiate the anatomical or topographical changes

produced,in the chest , by surgery or radiotherapy from neoplastic disease. In these cases, radiological investigation give us dou- btful patterns, while radioimmunodetection may put in avidence the presence of the tumour. In our experience the immunoscintigraphy clearly showed 9/10 lesions of the chest, 3/3 of the brain , 19/22 of the bones, and 4/4 of the abdomen (see Table 5 and Fig.5).

TABLE 5 Immunoscintigraphy After Surgical Treatment

ORGANS	$^{131}I+$	$^{111}In+$	TOTAL+
CHEST	2 / 3	7 / 7	9 / 10
NODES	--	1 / 2	1 / 2
BONE	2 / 2	17 / 20	19 / 22
BRAIN	1 / 1	2 / 2	3 / 3
ABDOMEN	1 / 1	3 / 3	4 / 4
TOTAL	6/7(85,7%)	30/34(88,2%)	36/41(87,8%)

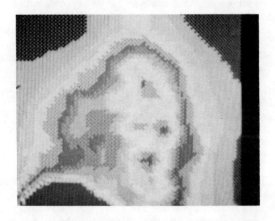

Fig. 5   Scintigraphic image of the chest

obtained , in anterior view, 72 hr after
administration of ^{111}In antiCEA reagent
(185 MBq). The patient was submitted ,15
months ago, to complete surgical removal of
right lung, for an epidermoid cancer. 9
months ago his serum CEA level resulted
higher (8 ng/ml) than normal range. The ra=
diological examinations resulted negative.
The immunoscintigraphy clearly showed an
hot spot in right hylar region and 3 sites
of uptake in the mediastinum. 6 months later a local recurrence and 3 lymph node me
tastases were found out by further inve =
stigations.

On these bases, a systematic employ of immunoscintigraphy in pa =
tients at high risk of relapse, may be suggested. This more exten
sive use of this new technique,will lead to an earlier detection
of small neoplastic deposits allowing more precocious treatments.

Radioimmunotherapy Results.
In 2 patients bearing a bulky and spread epidermoid lung cancer
(T_3 N_2 M_1) the antibody guided irradiation of the tumour , per =
formed by intravenous injection of radiolabelled MoAbs, did not
modify the progression of the neoplastic disease. 1 patient is dead
after 4 months. 1 patient is still alive but shows a significant
growth of the cancer after 8 months. More favourable results were
obtained in the 3rd patient. He was submitted, in March 1985 to
surgical removal of the right lung for an epidermoid carcinoma.
In July 1985 he developed a pleural recurrence that became irre-
sponsive to several chemotherapy and radiotherapy regimes. Since
the immunoscan, performed by intrapleural administration, showed a
strong uptake of MoAb on the tumour and the effective half life of
antibody resulted lenghtened we carried out an intrapleural radio
immunotherapy trial. We administered, 7 times, at monthly inter=
vals the aforementioned FO23C5 up to a total amount of 10 mg of
protein and 2590 MBq(70 mCi) of [131]I . The patient survived for
13 months,while his life expectance was of 3 months when the radio
immunotherapy was started. His pleural effusion decreased and the
malignant cells disappeared.

        DISCUSSION

Our studies , performed in a large group of patients, have shown
the high level both of sensitivity and specificity achievable by
means of radioimmunoscintigraphy. This technique is safe. It is
easily performed. It gives data regarding the antigenic feature of
lesions as well as local extension and   systemic spread of the
tumour. It appear very important , on the basis of the results so
far achieved, to evaluate the proper applications of this diagnostic tool for clinical purposes. The radioimmunolocalisation of
primary tumours,that are diagnosed by means of radiological and

bronchocoscopic examinations ,may be suggested mainly in those pa
tients with doubtful instrumental findings. The radioimmunoinve =
stigation of primary tumours, moreover, is useful in order to perform a complete evaluation of the patient before surgery. The detection of involved lymph nodes in the hylar region or in the me =
diastinum may help the surgeon to program the extension of the o=
peration. The diagnosis of systemic lesions, mainly when these are
undetectable by conventional methods, lead to chemotherapy or radio
therapy regimes, avoiding more aggressive procedures. When the immunoscintigraphy is carried out in patients already operated, the
outcomes achieved put in evidence the possibility to overcome the
limits of radiological examination who , in some cases, cannot distinguish the neoplastic recurrences from the fibrotic alterations.
The radioimmunolocalisation may be more usefully employed in pa =
tients who underwent to apparently complete surgical removal of the
tumour but who have an high probability of tumour relapse. These
"at high risk" patients are those with a large tumour ,whose diameter was about 2 cm, and with no more than 1 lymph node invol =
ved (T_2 N_1 M_0). The use of radioimmunodetection in this group of
patients which should be studied every 6-12 months,even in absence
of instrumental, serological or clinical findings, may lead to ear
lier diagnosis of local or distant metastases and indicate the
opportunity to start a more precocious treatment. Finally the radioimmunotherapy by means of radiolabelled MoAbs, presents actually many problems still unsolved. When the MoAbs are intravenously
injected, the percentage of radiopharmaceutical piked up by the tu
mour is about the 0,002% of administered dose. So that the radiation dose delivered to the neoplastic tissue is very low and does
not lead to a tumour shrinking effect. The intrapleural administration of MoAbs may, in part, overcome these limitations and represents an alternative route of injection more useful for therapeutical purposes. The favourable result obtained in a only patient
are similar to those achieved by means of intraperitoneal admini -
stration that we have carried out in ovarian (8) and colo-rectal
(7) cancer patients . In 60% of these patients, who were in advan
ced stage of disease, we obtained clinical and instrumental eviden
ce of complete (1) or partial remission of neoplastic disease. These results ,thus preliminary, look promising and suggest to broaden
these trials in order to collect more conclusive data.

REFERENCES

1. Buraggi G.L.,L.Callegaro,A.Turrin ,L.Gennari,E.Bombardieri,M.Ga
   sparini, G.Mariani,R.Doci,E.Regaglia and E.Sereni (1984). Immunoscintigraphy of colo-rectal carcinoma: remarks about an ongo-
   ing clinical trial. In H.A.E. Schmidt,D.E. Vaurama (Ed.),Nuklear-
   medizin , Schattauer Verlag Stuttgart,pp.629-632.

2. Chatal,J.F., J.C. Saccavini,P.Fumoleau,Douillard J.Y.,Curtet C.,
   Kremer M., Le Mevel B. and H.Koprowski (1984). Immunoscintigraphy of Colon Carcinoma.J.Nucl.Med.,25 ,307/314.

3. Epenetos A.A.,Snook D., Hooker G.,Begent R.,Durbin H.,Oliver
   R.T.D., Bodmer V.F. and Lavender J.P.(1985). Indium -111 la =
   belled Monoclonal Antibody to Placental Alkaline Phosphatase in
   the Detection of Neoplasms of Testis,Ovary,and Cervix.Lancet ii:
   350-353.

4. Garriguers H.J., W.Tilgen, J.Hellstrom,W.Franke and K.E.Hell-
   strom (1982). Detection of a Human Melanoma -Associated Antigen,
   p97,in Histological Sections of Primary Human Melanomas. J.Can-
   cer 29 , 511-515

5. Hammersmith Oncology Group (1984). Antibody - Guided Irradia =
   tion of Malignant Lesions: Three cases illustrating a new method
   of treatment. Lancet ii : 1441-1443

6. Hnatowich D.J.,W.W. Layne,R.Childs (1982). The preparation and
   labelling of DTPA coupled albumin. Int. J. Appl Radiat Isotop.
   33,327-332.

7. Humm J. L.(1986). Dosimetric Aspects of Radiolabeled Antibodies
   for Tumor Therapy. J.Nucl. Med.,27, 1490-1497.

8. Mariani G.,L.Callegaro,N.Mazzucca,E.Cecconato, M.Molea,M.Dovis,
   L.Fusani,G.Deleide,G.L.Buraggi and R.Bianchi (1984). Tissue Distribution of radiolabelled Anti-CEA Monoclonal Antibodies in
   man . Prot.Biol. Fluids .,32, 483-486.

9. Riva P.,G.Paganelli,G.Riceputi, G.Pasini,T.Panacea,G.Cacciaguer-
   ra and F.Giunchi (1986). In R.Hofer   and H.Bergmann (Ed) Ra-
   dioacktive Isotope in Klinik und Forschung,H.Egermann Vienna. pp
   403-407.

10 Sternberger L.A.(1979) The unlabelled peroxidase-antiperoxidase
   (PAP) method. John Wiley Sons.(Ed.) Immunocytochemistry,New York
   pp.104-169

11 Wahl ,R.L.,C.W. Parker and G.W.Philpott(1983). Improved radioi-
   maging and tumor localisation with monoclonal $F(ab')_2$. J. Nucl.
   Med. , 24, 316-325.

Laparoscopy in Small Cell Lung Cancer

G. Dagnini

Centro di Laparoscopia, Padova, Italy

Indifferentiated small cell lung cancer (microcytoma) has a marked tendency to spread precociously. The speed of cellular replication of the microcytoma is very high and can be compared to that of several forms of lymphoma (Livinston, 1980). That explains the remarkable sensibility of the tumor to radiation and chemotherapy, two types of treatment that have undoubtedly improved the prognosis (Oldham, 1980).

As for every tumor with a strong potential for metastasis, a rigorous staging is necessary before starting therapy, whether it is for prognostic purpose or to choose the most suitable program of treatment, which will include if it is possible, an operation.

Precise knowledge of the extension of the tumor is also important for evaluating the results of the therapeutic treatments whose standardization is not yet completely defined. It is, therefore, necessary to classify the patients precisely in order to correctly interprete and correlate the results obtained with various types of treatment. Clinical and instrumental staging is very important for a first selection of patients but there is no doubt that the resulting "limited" forms must be subjected as well to a "pathological" staging.

Laparoscopy, whose use is well-known for the staging of cancer of the esophagus and of the ovaries, of melanoblastomas and above all lymphomas, also responds well in microcytoma that has several characteristics common to systemic tumors (Dombernowsky, 1978; Dagnini, 1980; Hansen, 1978). The advent of imaging techniques has naturally reduced the number of laparoscopies indicated for the searching of tumoral metastases in the stomach.

Echography and CT scans are often capable of demonstrating the possible presence of metastasis, above all of an hepatic nature, of the tumor and of confirming this presence with a thin needle biopsy. In these cases, laparoscopy is obviously superfluous.

Our experience at the Padova Center is based on the observation of 138 cases of microcytoma gathered from 1981 on, in which, the preliminary clinical and instrumental exam revealed metastatic diffusion in 36 (Oldham, 1980). In the remaining 102 "negative" cases laparoscopy showed metastasis in 28 (23 of the liver, 3 of the peritoneum, 1 of the spleen and 1 of the ovary).

The laparoscopic percentage of positiveness and thus, stage advancement, is relevant. We must say that, being a question of retrospective investigation, the diagnostic potential of the echography was surely inferior when compared with current diagnostic methods and, at the time, we did not yet use thin needle biopsy. It must be remembered also that in our center, since 1984, the pre-laparoscopic echography has been proposed and then performed, with great advantages.

However the "false negatives" of the clinic staging of the microcytoma are relatively numerous and the very laparoscopic findings supply us with elements for the explanation of these mistakes.

Cases of hepatic metastasis of the microcytoma present characteristics that make if difficult for them to be spotted echographically because it is a question of: 1. small nodules which are little protruding (35%); 2. superficial patches (18%); 3. an apparently normal macroscopic picture with only a bioptical diagnosis (4,5%).

Moreover, echography does not "see" the extra-hepatic localizations (18%). The morphological analogies with the malignant lymphomas impose an identical staging for the microcytoma, that is, with laparoscopy and biopsy.

In spite of this, it is necessary to reckon with a certain number of "false negatives". The percentage of these is not evaluated because there is no possibility for abdominal surgical verification. Our false-negative figures are 5% in the staging of cancer of the esophagus (verified at surgery) and 15% approximately for HD lymphomas which resulted positive upon laparosplenectomy.

We must think, due to the previously mentioned analogies, that in microcytoma, the percentage of laparoscopic false negatives must approach that of the lymphomas more than that of cancer of the esophagus.

In spite of this, laparoscopy can be considered a very suitable means for completing the clinical staging of microcytoma.

Furthermore, it can be put to good use to follow the modifications of the lesions in the course of therapy (Follow-up). Echography can give important information on gross variations. Laparoscopy and biopsy consent more delicate findings and are even capable of documenting the eventual sterilization of the neoplastic focuses.

REFERENCES

Dagnini, G. (1980). Clinical Laparoscopy. Piccin Medical Books, Padova.

Dombernowsky, P., F. Hirsch, H. Hansen, and B. Hainau (1978). Peritoneoscopy in the staging of 190 patients with small-cell anaplastic carcinoma of the lung with special reference to subtyping. Cancer, 41, 2008-2012.

Hansen, H., P. Dombernowsky, and F. Hirsch (1978). Staging procedure and prognostic features in small-cell anaplastic bronchogenic carcinoma. Seminars in Oncology, 3, 280-287.

Livinston, R. (1980). Small-cell carcinoma of the lung. Blood, 4, 575-584.

Oldham, R.K., and F.A. Greco (1980). Small-cell lung cancer. A curable disease. Cancer Chemother. Pharmacol. 4, 173-177.

Patella, M., and coworkers (1984). Lo staging ed il follow-up laparoscopico del microcitoma del polmone. Gior. Ital. Endosc. Digest, 1, 25-30.

Tancini, G., and coworkers (1982). Impiego combinato della laparoscopia e della biopsia ossea nella determinazione dello stadio del carcinoma indifferenziato a piccole cellule del polmone. Valutazione di 116 casi consecutivi. Tumori, 68, 81-84.

The Clinical Importance of a Well Designed Clinical, Biochemical and Instrumental Follow-up Program

M. Clavel*, P. Rebattu* and V. Trillet†

*Centre Léon Bérard, Lyon;
†Hôpital Cardio-Vasculaire et Pneumologique,
Lyon, France

ABSTRACT

Various clinical trials claim for higher response rate and longer survival of SCLC patients. Heterogeneity of classification and prognostic factors make uneasy the evaluation of the results. Better results may be only better patients' selection.

KEYWORDS

Staging, restaging, prognostic factors.

INTRODUCTION

The overall prognosis of small cell lung cancer (S.C.L.C.) patients remains very poor. In contrast, many treatments such as chemotherapy and radiotherapy are able to give a high response rate. Furthermore, if surgery was claimed to be useless for the last decades, this treatment in a highly selected subset of patients should be reconsidered.
In spite of high response rate, no real improvement is demonstrated in term of cure rate, and the long term survival after three years is still minimal. Multimodality treatments are becoming the standard procedures for non metastatic patients, but the choice of the initial treatment is queering : initial chemotherapy followed by radiotherapy ? chemotherapy and radiotherapy in a sandwich alternating procedure, place of an initial surgery.
Many trials are published but the conclusions are limited because it is very difficult to compare the various treated populations.
While chemotherapy is improving, prognostic factors are being well known either concerning the tumor itself or concerning the patient bearing tumor. The improvements of the treatment and a definite consensus for the treatment are only possible from comparative conclusive trials.
To compare the response rates in various trials means no difference in patients accrual and in criteria of eligibility. It is why a consensus initial work up is required.
To compare the median times of response, disease-free survival and overall survival means no difference in the follow-up procedures.
The initial staging, the follow-up procedures and a post-treatment staging (restaging) are the bases for a well designed follow-up program.

THE INITIAL STAGING : WHY ?

In S.C.L.C., systemic chemotherapy is the main treatment, regardless of the stage. Therefore, the design of an optimal plan of therapy is not closely dependent on accurate assessment of tumor dissemination except for the very small group of patients who are eligible for surgical resection.

Considering the well-known prognostic factors in this disease, most of them such as intra-thoracic vs extensive disease, initial performance status, and weight loss are obviously related to the tumor burden and the number of metastatic sites. The role of initial staging is therefore to distinguish not only non metastatic from metastatic patients (who will usually not require local treatment), but also to evaluate the response after initial treatment.

Some localizations may require an individual therapeutic decision when discovered, such as CNS involvement where local irradiation may be recommanded as first line therapy even when the tumor is clinically asymptomatic.

As far as treatment tolerance is concerned, some metastatic sites may increase the toxicity and therefore may require dose adaptation, for instance BM involvement or hepatic dysfunction due to liver metastases.

At last, evaluation of treatment efficiency is mainly based on the comparison between initial and residual tumor volume after therapy, that is, between initial staging and restaging at the end of the treatment program.

THE INITIAL STAGING : HOW ?

The staging system for primary lung cancer defined by the American Joint Committee (AJC) for Staging and Results Reporting is based on the TNM classification. The usefulness of this system is to predict surgical resectability when applied to SCLC, only a small subset of patients (about 10 %) have operable (stage I or stage II) disease. Therefore, the TNM system fails to provide useful information for the majority of S.C.L.C. patients.

An alternative and widely applied staging system is that of the Veterans Administration Lung Cancer Study Group, intented to separate patients whose disease could or could not be encompassed in a single radiation field. Thus, most of the treatments programs are based on the classification between 2 sub groups : limited (to the thorax) and extensive disease. Limited disease includes involvement of one hemithorax with or without ipsilateral supra-clavicular lymph nodes and pleura. This lack of homogeneity in the classification for one series to an other requires a very carefull study of the definition of "limited" and "extensive" patients before comparing treatment results in the litterature.

Intra-thoracic dissemination of the tumor is usually wide, mediastinal lymph nodes being easily detectable on a standard chest X ray in most cases. This procedure also provides adequate assessment of pleural effusion although cytological examination is necessary since it is positive in only 53 % of the patients. X-ray tomography generally provides little additional information. CT scan enables an estimate of tumor volume, but it should not be considered a routine requirement because it may lead to too many false positive findings. Bronchoscopy is very useful in establishing the histo-logical diagnosis and describing the initial endobronchial extension ; mediastinoscopy is required for histological diagnosis only when the tumor is not accessible to the bronchoscopy. It is too early to know whether more sophisticated techniques such as IRM will provide more informations than the routine procedures. Nevertheless one must keep in mind that, as far as initial thoracic staging is concerned, only the presence or absence of pleural or supraclavicular spread determines both the treatment program and the prognosis. That is why the only procedures recommended as necessary in the last international workshop on S.C.L.C. are clinical examination, chest X-ray and fiberoptic bronchoscopy.

According to the litterature (IHDE and HANSEN have collected 8 series with a total of 734 patients), the most commonly involved organs are bone (19 to 38 %), liver (18 to 34 %), lymph nodes (16 to 55 %), bone marrow (11 to 47 %), brain (O to 14 %), soft tissue (3 to 11 %) and opposite lung (7-8 %).

Radionucleide bone scanning is a sensitive but relatively non-specific technique for assessing bone involvement. Isolated abnormalities, in the context of a degenerative joint disease should be confirmed in these cases by X-ray. Although a large number of false positive results are found with this method, it is still used as a routine evaluation procedure by a majority of authors since it is the only one available for bone metas-tases assessment.

Non specific abnormalities are frequently reported with radionucleide scanning and this method cannot be used as a guide for fine needle aspiration, cytological and/or histological examination of liver metastases may be done with the use of ultrasonography or CT scanning (specificity 92 %, sensitivity 64 % in 66 patients who subsequently underwent peritoneoscopy). Despite these recent technological developments, staging of the liver is still problematic, and non of them is recommended as a routine procedure. From a biological point of view, serum alkaline phosphatases and LDH are unconstantly elevated, SGOT has a reasonnable sensitivity but it is only elevated in 60 % of the patients with liver metastases.

The common practice to detect bone marrow involvement is the use of unilateral crest marrow aspiration and biopsy. Bilateral biopsies are often not performed although they rise the positive yield to about 30 % ; the detection of abnormal cells in the marrow is now possible with the use of monoclonal antibodies (MOC-1, TFS-2 or SM1 for instance) on fresh blood samples, and some involvements which were undetectable with standard cytological and histological techniques have been shown.

CT scanning is superior to scintigraphy of the brain and may result in early diagnosis of asymptomatic cases, and we have already mentionned the therapeutic implication of such a finding, but new high-resolution gamma cameras could improve the radionucleide technique. Lumbar puncture is indicated only when a meningeal involvement is clinically suspected. CT scan of the abdomen is usefull for the detection of retroperitoneal metastases, especially adrenal glands which now appear to be a common metastatic site.

As a conclusion, 4 important points are to be mentionned :
a) based on these results, a consensus from the workshop on S.C.L.C. in 1983 recommended the following procedure as routine tests at the time of diagnosis : chest X-ray, bronchoscopy, bone marrow aspiration and biopsy, and fine needle of any skin or lymph node and pleural effusion.
b) since the treatment is only defined by the presence or absence of extra-thoracic disease, the critical situation is the following : a single metastatic site is suspected, based on the result of a test which sensitivity and specificity are known to be low. In this case where a patient might not benefit of an effective modality of treatment - namely radiotherapy - because of a false-positive test, we believe that as many tests as possible should be repeated and compared, and that the role of fine needle aspirations under US or CT control is predominant. A very interesting study (HOLOYE) has recently shown that among 50 patients, bone scan was the only abnormal test in 2 cases, liver-spleen radionucleide scan and CT scan of the abdomen in 4 cases, and bone marrow aspiration in 4 cases. Considering the high level of false positive results with bone scan when the patients are asymptomatic, the authors concluded that this procedure could be deleted from the initial staging.
c) the cost and time consuming aspects of most of the techniques we have described make them irrelevant and even dangerous when they increase the time from diagnosis to the treatment without modifying the stage, the therapeutic decision, or the prognosis of an individual patient, unless they are necessary for improving the knowledge of the disease.
d) the last aspect of the pre-therapeutic staging is its use for the follow-up and evaluation of response after completion of the treatment.

THE FOLLOW-UP PROCEDURES

To compare the clinical trials results in term of time to response, time to recurrence, time of response, time of disease-free survival and survival, the same methods should be used for calculation.

So the rythm of examination, the techniques of examination, should be previously established and published.

On a methodologic point, it is well known that closer is the follow-up, shorter is the delay between two consecutive evaluation, longer is the duration of response or survival. In the situation of a carefully determined clinical trial, there is no doubt that a very strict clinical and biological assessment is necessary in order to evaluate the results in the case of an individual patient, and because of the lack of efficiency of the treatments when the relapse occurs, a 6 months to 6 months follow-up might be sufficient.

THE RESTAGING

As for many other tumors from various site and pathology, the response to treatment is clearly shown to be due of the major prognostic factor.

The response to treatment is done by comparison of restaging data and initial data. For instance, bone scanning which does not appear as necessary for the diagnosis, may serve as a usefull baseline for subsequent examinations and thoracic CT scan enables to evaluate minimal residual disease (but cannot distinguish between necrotic or evolutive tumor mass). It is to be mentionned that bronchoscopy is not universally employed for restaging and it is important in reading the litterature to note whether criterias for complete tumor response included bronchoscopic confirmation.

The quality of response is also important to be noted since only complete responders may have the chance to be cured.

Regardless of the non-responders who are usually rapidly progressive and poor short-term prognostic patients, the aim of this evaluation is to separate CR from PR patients. But one can wonder about the validity of such a re-assessment since the majority of the patients relapse within a few months, most of the so-called CRs are probably PRs with minimal residual disease, undetectable with our imaging methods. Nevertheless, the need for such a distinction between CR and PR is understandable since it usually implies a different therapeutic decision : in the case of complete remission an alternative between further abstention or additional treatment whatever it is called "maintenance", "consolidation", "intensification" or prophylaxy on a "sanctuary" ; in the case of partial response, a switch to a different but probably palliative treatment modality. Surgical re-staging is rarely used although it is the best modality of local evaluation and treatment macroscopic and histologic re-assessment and eventually tumor "debulking".

Two different clinical situations in regard of the importance of a clinical, biochemical and instrumental follow-up program are to be considered :

1 - S.C.L.C. routine treatment. In a routine situation a minimal work-up is sufficient and a general consensus for an initial work-up is well established before treatment starts. 2 - In clinical research situation, no initial work-up limitation is standardized and so new prognostic factors or clinical subsets may appear.

In this situation, definitions of limited or extensive disease should be very precise and accurate as for the evaluation of complete response. This evaluation should require more specific data including aspiration cytology when extrathoracic disease is known.

Radiotherapy in Small Cell Lung Cancer

M. Cappellini, S. M. Magrini and R. Mungai

U.O. di Radioterapia, Unità Sanitaria Locale 10/D,
Policinico Careggi, Viale Morgagni, 50134 Firenze, Italy

ABSTRACT

The aim of the present review is to evaluate radiotherapy role in the treatment
of small cell lung cancer (SCLC). Total dose, fractionation, volumes and different ways for integrating radiotherapy and chemotherapy are discussed, with
particular reference to the role of palliative, radical and systemic
radiotherapy.

KEY WORDS

Lung cancer, SCLC, Radiobiology, Radiotherapy, Combined Modality Treatment.

INTRODUCTION

Although in patients with small cell lung cancer short term survival has increased with the introduction of new treatment modalities, so far there hasn't
been a corresponding improvement in long-term survival, as evidenced in the
following table.

TABLE 1   Short and Long Term Survival in Patients with "Limited Disease" SCLC
According to Different Treatment Modalities (Surgery not Included) 1972-1985.

Treatment Modality	% Survival (yrs) 1	2	3	4	5	>5	Year of Report	Pts	Follow-up min.	Ref.
RT only	*	19	11	4				1972	27	3 yrs	Carr, D.T.
RT only	*	22	10			4	4	1973	73	10 yrs	Fox, W.
RT only	*	18	5	3				1981	121	3 yrs	Bleehen, N.M.
CT only	*	5	0					1975	31	–	Laing, A.H.
CT only	*	35	10	10				1985	37	9-77 mos	Lichter, A.S.
RT + CT	*	23	6	6				1972	31	3 yrs	Carr, D.T.
RT + CT	*	34	9	4				1981	115	3 yrs	Bleehen, N.M.
RT + CT						11		1984	118	8 yrs	Livingston, R.B.
RT + CT	*	65	35	35	20			1985	37	9-77 mos	Lichter, A.S.
RT + CT						11		1985	103	5 yrs	Johnson, B.E.

RT = Radiotherapy   CT = Chemotherapy   * Randomized Studies.

The table shows an improvement of 30-40% in the 1 year survival, over the last 15 years, against only about a 5% increase in long-term survival. It should be noted that the latter difference in percentage refers to the "tail" of the survival curves and therefore it is statistically less significant. Also, in recent controlled studies, there has been a tendency to select patients with better performance status. The data reported in the table refer to favourably selected patients, who belonged to the "limited disease" group according to the Veterans Administration Lung Cancer Study Group (VALCSG) classification. Moreover, the hope that aggressive radiochemotherapy may cure a significant number of these patients (pts) has led to a more accurate staging. As mentioned by Ihde (1981) this may apparently improve results in the two groups defined by VALCSG and taken individually, without any actual improvement in the prognosis of both groups. In fact, those cases with early distant metastases, detected with a more accurate staging, show longer survival: hence an apparent improvement of prognosis in the group with extended disease. On the other hand, pts with worse prognosis will thus be ruled out from the limited disease group. To conclude: the different types of locoregional therapy are hardly ever successful for the early appearance of distant metastases which cannot be prevented with available systemic treatments, even in the smaller group of patients (20-30%) with limited disease.

SCLC STAGING FROM A RADIOTHERAPIST'S POINT OF VIEW

Despite what is mentioned above, the Authors feel that a more accurate staging can be very useful in SCLC pts for two main reason: a) it allows selection of pts who may benefit from aggressive treatment aiming at cure. Patients with truly limited disease (T_1 T_2 N_0 M_0 as per American Joint Committee for End Results Reporting and Staging - AJC) may survive 5 years after radical surgery in 30-40% of cases (Cataldo, 1987; George, 1986). Also the results presented at this Congress evidence an increase in long-term survival after radical surgery: 20% - 30% - 50% parallel to the increase, in the same series, in the percentage of pts with stage I (AJC): 30% - 45% - 55%. The same approach can be applied to radical radiotherapy, which has prouved capable of obtaining a modest but reproducible percentage of long-term cures in selected pts; b) accurate staging allows clear appreciation of the effectiveness of therapy if the initially positive sites are systematically reinvestigated after therapy with the same diagnostic tools. This particularly important assumption is confirmed by the complete remission radiologically observed after chemotherapy in those pts who still present endobronchial disease at bronchoscopy (Ihde 1981). These data are important for a correct evaluation of the role of radiotherapy in combined treatments. It is not surprising, therefore, that the suggestion of using TNM also in SCLC staging, initially put forward by surgeons (Carr, 1983) has recently been adopted also by radiotherapists (Byhardt, 1986). A TNM-like classification therefore seems to be able to define three prognosis subgroups -instead of two, as in VALCSG classification. A classification as proposed by Byhardt, for instance, helps to select those pts who better benefit from radiotherapy, even when chemotherapy is the mainstay of treatment.

SOME BIOLOGICAL AND RADIOBIOLOGICAL ISSUES

The peculiar natural history of SCLC makes research in its biology - peculiar in itself - extremely interesting. However, although a better understanding of the biology of SCLC may lead to greater chances of cure, at the moment the radiotherapist is interested in a less ambitious objective. The questions to be answered are essentially two: a) are SCLC biological characteristics such as to suggest using total doses very different from those usually employed in other types of lung cancer? In other words, can we talk about greater radio-curability, besides greater SCLC radioresponsiveness, with respect to other lung malignancies and from a local control point of view? b) is the disease marked sensitiveness to chemotherapy equivalent to high curability of the disease with this modality or is radiotherapy necessary to consolidate results? If so, optimal total and fractional doses should be known together with the best way to integrate with chemotherapy, when this is used. An answer to the first question may be found in the reports from the literature on the various parameters used to evaluate tumor radiosensitivity, with particular reference to SCLC, according to the following table.

TABLE 2 Radiosensitivity Determinants

A - "INBORN" CHARACTERISTICS OF CELL RESPONSE TO IRRADIATION
- "Intrinsic" radiosensitivity (D_0, SF_2, α);
- "Intrinsic" radioresistance (N, "recovery ratio", PLDR)

B - FACTORS MODIFYING "IN VIVO" CELL RESPONSE TO IRRADIATION
- Tumor "structural" characteristics (necrosis, hypoxia);
- Tumor "kinetic" characteristics (doubling time, label-ling index, lenght of cell cycle, distribution in cell cycle phases)
- Heterogeneity of cell subpopulations forming the tumor.

"Inborn" Characteristics of Cell Response to Irradiation

"Intrinsic" radiosensitivity. D_0 obtained in vitro with many cell lines from different tumors are substantially similar, i. e., an analysis of this para-meter does not show a significant difference in SCLC intrinsic radiosensitiv-ity in culture with respect to other lung tumors and other malignancies - as reported in the following table.

TABLE 3 D_0 of Several Tumor-Derived Cell Lines Irradiated "in vitro"

Data from Russo (1985), Malaise (1986), Duchesne (1986)

Tumor	Cell lines studied	D_0 (Gy) Mean (Range)
SCLC	5	1.10 (0.51-1.40)
SCLC	5	1.21 (0.89-1.59)
SCLC	6	1.51 (-)
ADENOCA. LUNG	2	1.51 (1.13-1.90)
ADENOCA. LUNG	2	1.81 (1.81-1.82)
EPID. CARCINOMA LUNG	5	1.59 (1.28-1.84)
LARGE CELL CARCINOMA LUNG	1	1.48 (-)
MEDULLOBLASTOMA	2	1.32 (1.31-1.35)
OSTEOSARCOMA	2	1.40 (1.35-1.45)
MELANOMA	3	1.34 (1.00-1.51)
MELANOMA	19	1.04 (-)

A more recent method proposed by Fertil (1981) and Deacon (1984) for evaluating the intrinsic radiosensitivity of the tumors is based on the concept that the

surviving fraction after 2 Gy (SF_2) is indicative - also clinically - of the
radiosensitivity of the tumor the irradiated cell line derives from. These
Authors report a progressive increase in mean SF_2 from the group of tumors
more clinically radiosensitive to that of the more radioresistant ones. The
differences between the SF_2 of the cell lines forming each group, however,
are sometimes greater than the differences between the mean SF_2 of the various
groups. In Deacon's report too, mean SF_2 is hardly more than double, passing
from the more radiosensitive to the more radioresistant group (0.19 - 0.52).
But a difference of the same order is observed between the cell lines derived
from SCLC (0.10 - 0.20). A more recent report from the same Authors (Duchesne,
1986) specifically analyses the cell lines derived from lung tumors with different histotype. The five "pure" SCLC lines obtained by these Authors show
a 0.33 mean SF_2 (0.22 - 0.45 range) - a little higher, therefore, than the
one mentioned above. The four lines derived from lung tumors with different
histotype seem to have mean SF_2 which are slightly higher but with ample range
(0.30 - 0.81). Unfortunately, for each of the other lung cancer histotypes,
the number of cell lines analysed with reference to SF_2 and reported is low
with respect to the number of lines obtained from SCLC and other human tumors
- melanoma for instance.
Recently, Malaise (1986) and other Authors (Thames, 1986) have revised the
use of SF_2 as an indicator of the intrinsic radiosensitivity of human tumors
and proposed to add to it other parameters which would better describe the
initial slope of the survival curve of the "in vitro" irradiated cells. These
parameters - α value, $\overline{D}$, etc. - derive from the more recent mathematic models
used to describe the biphase trend of the survival curve. These parameters
do not seem to have yielded results different from the previous ones.

Intrinsic radioresistance. Those Authors who have focused their attention on
the causes of intrinsic radioresistance have shown a different attitude as
regards the characterization of the first portion of the survival curve of
irradiated cells.
The value of the extrapolation number ($\underline{N}$) can be regarded as a measure of the
amplitude of the shoulder and consequently of the ability of the cell to repair
sublethal damage (SLD). The following table reports mean values for different
cell lines derived from SCLC and various other human tumors and irradiated
"in vitro". These values should express the different ability to accumulate
SLD of the different cell lines.

TABLE 4 N Values of "In Vitro" - Irradiated Human Tumor - Derived Cell Lines

Data from Russo (1985), Malaise (1986), Duchesne (1986)

Tumor	Cell lines	N - Mean (Range)
SCLC	5	1.66 (1.00-3.30)
SCLC	6	1.80 (-)
SCLC	5	1.95 (1.51-2.75)
ADENOCA. LUNG	2	2.50 (2.00-3.00)
ADENOCA. LUNG	2	1.66 (1.34-1.99)
EPID. CARCINOMA	5	1.66 (1.50-2.10)
MEDULLOBLASTOMA	2	2.00 (1.80-2.20)
MELANOMA	3	14.50 (2.00-40.0)
MELANOMA	19	73.00 (-)

The above remarks regarding D_0 are true for this parameter too, apart from
the high N value of the melanoma - derived cell lines; this does not seem,
therefore, to evidence a particular radiosensitivity of SCLC.

Another method for measuring the ability to repair SLD is that of establishing the ratio (recovery ratio, RR) between the survival fractions (SF) of the cell lines irradiated with the same dose in two fractions or in single fraction, respectively. With this method, Duchesne (1986) has not found significant differences in the ability to repair SLD, between the six lines derived from lung malignancies with different histotype and including also lines derived from SCLC. More recently, other experimental parameters have been introduced, also as regards intrinsic radioresistance, for a better characterization of cell lines. For instance, Weichselbaum (1986) and others have recently correlated the radioresistance of different cell lines with their ability to repair potentially lethal damage (PLD). This type of damage appears when the cells - irradiated in relatively unfavourable culture conditions - are rapidly transferred into subculture after exposure. If the cells are not immediately transferred after irradiation the damage can be repaired. PLD repair (PLDR) would seem to be a particularly interesting phenomenon as it would occur in conditions similar to those of tumor cells "in vivo": low pH, scarce availability of O_2 and nutrients. However, PLDR does not seem to be so regularly different in the different tumor cell lines (Duchesne, 1986; Weichselbaum, 1986) as to allow a clear distinction between radiosensitive and radioresistant tumors.

Factors Modifying Intrinsic Radiosensitivity "In Vivo"

The cells forming a particular tissue are not interindependent: they form a complex structure having a delicate equilibrium between cell proliferation and death. When studying radiation-induced damage in a tissue we cannot therefore consider cell death only as quantified by survival curves: also the structure organization (vascularization, for instance) must be considered together with the tissue proliferation kinetics. This is true for both healthy and neoplastic tissues. The latter, moreover, present, almost always, cell subpopulations with different biological and radiobiological characteristics; i.e., they have strongly heterogeneous components. This complicates the investigation of their "in vivo" response to radiation and its determining factors. Many data, in fact, confirm the difference between the "in vitro" and "in vivo" response to radiation for various tumors (Malaise, 1986). Duchesne data (1986) specifically refer to lung tumors and SCLC and show an increase in SF_2 and radioresistance when the tumor is irradiated "in vivo". It is therefore important to find out the conditions which underlie this greater "in vivo" radioresistance.

Tumor "structural" characteristics. Among the structural causes of "in vivo" radioresistance should be included a fraction of hypoxic cells which cannot, however, be measured directly without great difficulties (Denekamp, 1983; Kallman, 1986). The hypoxic fraction as calculated by Duchesne (1986) for 4 lines derived from SCLC and irradiated "in vivo" - as xenografts - or "in vitro" - as spheroids about half a millimeter in diameter - was in the order of 20-30%. Hypoxic cells seems to be localized near the margins of the necrotic areas. It is important to note, therefore, that most pathological studies report the presence of large necrotic areas in SCLC (Carter, 1980; Cohen, 1978).
To conclude: in SCLC, the structure of neoplastic tissue and in particular its vascularisation do not seem such as to lead to particular radiocurability.

Tumor "kinetic" characteristics. Historically, one of the first parameters assessed to define the modality of tumor growth was doubling time (DT) which can be measured in different ways. In metastases and tumors of the lungs this is done by means of chest X-rays taken at different time intervals after diagnosis. This is the subject of many reports, which refer to cases which were not treated for different reasons. Assuming that fast growing tumors - with shorter DT - better respond to radio-chemotherapy than tumors with long DT, efforts have been made to demonstrate that the length of DT for SCLC is shorter than in other lung tumors. If the data available on this subject are accurately examined, it can be observed, however, that the values estimated for SCLC have been increasing in parallel to the increase in the number of observations.

TABLE 5 Radiological Doubling Time Values in SCLC

Data from Chahinian, 1972; Meyer, 1973; Straus, 1974; Tubiana, 1977; Brigham, 1978

Mean (days)	Range (days)	Cases	Year of the report
23.5	23 - 24	2	1973
39	17 - 71	3	1972
33	-	5	1974
68	17 - 264	46	1977
91	25 - 160	12	1978

Considering the largest series (Shackney, 1978; Straus, 1983), therefore, a mean DT can be observed which is fully comparable to that of other lung tumors with the exception of adenocarcinoma, which, as well known, has a markedly longer mean DT. Even if we assume that DT is significantly shorter in SCLC than in other lung tumors, there is still to demonstrate that DT is actually correlated with radiocurability. Breur (1966) was one of the first Authors to hypothesize a relationship between DT and radioresponsiveness. In his series of 16 pts with lung metastases a more rapid and complete volume reduction of the metastatic masses after irradiation was obtained when DT was shorter. Breur himself, however, makes it clear that although showing a less marked and rapid volume reduction, metastatic masses regrow more slowly when DT is longer. A greater volume reduction in neoplastic masses seems therefore to be rapidly cancelled for the more intense proliferative activity of the survived tumor cells. Only when the tumor does not regrows after irradiation-however simplistic this parameter may sound - can we say that the tumor is radiocurable (Breur, 1966; Malaise, 1972). The information from the study of DT both before and after radiotherapy shift our interest towards more sensitive parameters for the study of tumor kinetics. For SCLC in particular it would be interesting to explain the discrepancy between the rapid response to radiotherapy and chemotherapy, which is frequently observed and the equally frequent treatment failures. DT describes the volume growth of the neoplasm as a whole but not the behaviour of the different cell components of the tumor itself. They are essentially three: clonogenic, quiescent and end stage cells. With their proliferation, the first are responsible for the growth of the tumor; the second may be led to replicate by particular "environmental" stimuli. The end stage cells are absolutely incapable of replication and are doomed to be progressively eliminated from the tumor mass. The cell loss factor, in fact, indicates the percentage of cells originated from the clonogens and doomed to die without replicating. This factor may go up to 99% in many human carcinomas (Fowler, 1986). It is therefore particularly interesting to get to know the potential doubling time (T pot) which indicates the time necessary for a tumor to double its volume if it consisted only of clonogens and quiescent cells. T pot cannot be calculated directly. It is however possible to measure the labelling index (LI), i.e., the percentage of cells of a given tumor which are "labelled" by the tritiated thymidine they were administered and which therefore are in S phase. If we assume that the cell loss factor is very high in human tumors an approximate evaluation of T pot is possible and the resulting values will be lower than DT. Fowler (1986), for example, estimates that LI over 10-15% are associated with 5 day or shorter T pot. Short T pot and high LI are peculiar to malignancies characterized, also clinically, by rapid growth (Malaise, 1973). A recent survey (Straus, 1983) of LI values in lung cancers with different histotypes seem to demonstrate that the SCLC has a relatively high LI (16%) in comparison to LI of other lung tumors (3-10%). Kerr (1984) practically confirms these conclusions. In 17 out of the 27 pts investigated, the comparison of DT with calculated T pot, with cell loss factor and with LI was possible. The marked discrepancy observed between DT and T pot values can be explained by a cell loss factor always above 70% and over 90% in those cases with indifferentiated hystotype. In the two cases with SCLC 98% and 90% cell loss factors corresponded to 2.2 and 2.5 day T pot for a 22.5% and 20.3% LI respectively. Tumors like SCLC, with shorter T pot and therefore high mitotic rhythm, can respond to irradiation with a rapid volume reduction. In other words, the radioresponsiveness of the tumor is high as happens with all tissues, healthy or not, with high mitotic rhythm. Despite all this, in the absence of high intrinsic radiosensitivity and because of the prompt repopulation which may occur from the survived clonogens, a tumor of this kind cannot be termed radiocurable. Tubiana (1984) has demonstrated that higher LI associates with greater risk of local relapse and distant dissemination. Other Authors have come to the same conclusions (Peters, 1986; Silvestrini, 1985). It should be noted, in passing and in relation to what will be said later about SCLC heterogeneity, that in tumors with high LI a greater "genetic instability" is observed, which more easily leads to the emerging of "variant" cell lines, resistent to different therapeutic agents (Tubiana, 1986). We can therefore quote Peters (1982): "... there is no doubt that prompt initial regression is not a prerequisite for cure... in the final analysis, the rate of regression of a tumor following irradiation is of much less consequence than whether it is ultimately controlled". The following definition of radioresistance is therefore derived: "... A tumor is clinically radioresistant if it regrows within the irradiated region, regardless of its rate of regression". For this reason we can affirm, with reference to SCLC too, that: "... a rapid tumor regression should not lead to a reduction of the planned dose. It should be remembered that the radiation dose which induces a complete clinical remission is equal to only one third of the dose required to control the tumor" (Tubiana, 1983).

Tumor heterogeneity. As well known, the heterogeneity of cell populations forming a tumor is, radiobiologically, a radioresistance factor for different reasons, which are valid at least theoretically. If cell populations forming a tumor are heterogeneous, one of them could show higher intrinsic radioresistance. The heterogeneity of a tumor is tied to the "progression" towards a more malignant phenotype of the only clone which initially constitutes the tumor. As this occurs mostly in the primary tumor, it is here that more frequent is the presence of many different clones, some of which are more radioresistant. Tumor heterogeneity may also result into greater drug resistance. It follows that the site with greater risk of relapse after chemotherapy in SCLC is the primary one; here, association with radiotherapy should theoretically be more useful.

Flow cytofluorometry (FCM) makes it possible to detect the fraction of cells in S phase, in tumor and non-tumor cell populations. As this method is based, as well known, on the determination of DNA content, it also makes it possible to detect the presence of aneuploid cells and possibly of subpopulations with a different degree of aneuploidy, i.e., of different neoplastic clones in samples from the same tumor. The percentage of actively proliferating cells in SCLC (17%), evaluated with this method (Raber, 1980) compares with that from LI investigations (11-23%). The most interesting feature, however, is the datum on multiclonality - over one third of the tumors investigated includes more than one neoplastic clone (Mauro, 1986; Vindelov, 1980). This method, therefore, shows marked heterogeneity of SCLC and other lung tumors. By means of serial FCM evaluations in the same patient Vindelov (1980) has observed two neoplastic clones before any treatment; the elimination of one clone after chemotherapy; complete remission after radiotherapy started at that point. The relapse observed in this case might be correlated, speculatively, with the emergence of a third neoplastic clone, considering that distinct subpopulations are not detected with FCM when they are not over 5% of neoplastic cells (Straus, 1983). FCM is interesting, theoretically so far, as a rapid, reproducible method to define, in each individual patient, those biological characteristics of the tumor which are important for the treatment. Other experimental methods are available to demonstrate the heterogeneity of lung tumors and of SCLC in particular. Different clones within cell lines from the same tumor have been demonstrated - for SCLC - with monoclonal antibodies specific for antigenic determinants of tumor cells (Olsson, 1984). It is particularly interesting to note that cell lines derived from SCLC and cultured long enough, loose some of their biochemical characteristics, although the chromosomic alteration typical of this tumor is preserved (Whang-Peng, 1982). At the same time their morphology becames typically "large-celled". This "clonal evolution" is accompanied by the acquisition of a particular radioresistance, indipendently demonstrated by different Authors (Carney, 1983; Goodwin, 1982). Clinical extrapolation of this type of experimental results is obviously rather risky. However, if we accept a parallel between the appearance of large-celled "variant" lines "in vitro" and small- and large-celled tumors (SCLC-v or "variant") "in vivo", we might drow some temporary conclusions. In fact, SCLC-v does not seem to respond so well to chemo-radiotherapy clinically (Hirsch, 1983; Matthews, 1981). To conclude, vast areas of necrotic - and very likely hypoxic - tissue, a large fraction of rapidly proliferating cells and the marked heterogeneity of its cell constituents, together with an intrinsic radiosensitivity not much above that of other lung tumors, make SCLC quite radioresistant. Since a small portion of pts are cured with radiotherapy only and since chemotherapy frequently fails to sterilize the primary tumor, which is controlled by associated radiotherapy, this should be given in high total dose. The radiation tolerance of the various critical organs - particularly of the lungs - should therefore be taken into account.

RADIOTHERAPY IN SCLC: TOTAL DOSES, FRACTIONATION, TREATMENT TECHNIQUES. BIOLOGICAL BASIS AND THEIR CLINICAL IMPLICATIONS.

The following table shows the different uses of radiotherapy in the treatment of SCLC. Roughly, there are four types of employment: a) radical treatment - as sole modality or associated with others -; b) palliative and/or symptomatic treatment; c) as a "systemic" treatment (half-and total-body irradiation); d) prophylactic treatment of sites not easily reached by drugs. In individual clinical situations the necessary total dose and fractionation may vary widely, like the treated volume, also for the different extension of the tumor and for the different anatomic site to be irradiated.

TABLE 6 Radiotherapy in SCLC: Present and "Historical" Possibilities

A. AS PRIMARY TREATMENT
   - Radical radiotherapy only;

B. ASSOCIATED WITH OTHER MODALITIES
   - Radiotherapy associated with chemotherapy;
   - Pre-and postoperative radiotherapy;
   - Prophylactical brain irradiation (PBI);
   - Prophylactical spinal cord irradiation;
   - Prophylactical upper hemiabdomen irradiation;

C. AS "SYSTEMIC" TREATMENT
    - Half-body irradiation;
    - Sequential hemibody irradiation;
    - Total body irradiation;
D. AS SYMPTOMATIC AND PALLIATIVE TREATMENT

In each of these situations, to the above-mentioned causes of radioresistance should be added the need to spare the healthy adjacent tissues.
Naturally, the radiotherapist's interest focuses on the irradiation of the primary, which, when the tumor is truly limited, often has a radical aim and is frequently associated with chemotherapy.
The lung tissue is particularly sensitive to irradiation. According to Rubin (1972) the dose capable of inducing severe clinical complications in 25-50% of cases is about 60 Gy, when irradiation is carried out with conventional fractionation on a lung volume equivalent to a lobe. A much lower dose (40 Gy) is sufficient to cause radiologically evident fibrosis in almost all cases (Cionini, 1974; Libshitz, 1973). Irradiating large volumes with the same dose obviously has more severe clinical consequences. Doses slightly over 20 Gy with conventional fractionation involve a high risk of treatment-related fatalities, when the whole lung volume is exposed. Higher than 2 Gy fractional doses produce a more marked "late" lung damage (fibrosis) with equal "acute" damage . Therefore, the use of small fractional doses on volumes as limited as possible - thanks to the use of personalized fields, "coning down technique", etc. - contributes to improve therapeutic index.
Let us now consider the clinical evidence which seems to demonstrate the advantage of using high total doses, small fractional doses and limited volumes in the radical treatment of SCLC.
The need to treat SCLC with high doses can be clinically demonstrated in three ways: a) if those treated in this way prevail among long survivors; b) if the use of high doses induces complete remissions (CR) or local disease control in higher number of cases, considering that long survivors have almost always responded to primary treatment with CR; c) finally, with autoptic studies. As early as 1973, Fox and Scadding reported three cured cases out of a series of 62 pts treated with radical radiotherapy only with minimum ten-year follow-up. Two of the survived pts had received doses in the order of 50 Gy and more. Peschel (1981) observed that 12 of the 17 pts survived for over 2 years after treatment out of 244 treated for SCLC were relapse-free 24 months after treatment. Four of these 12 relapsed later on. 3 died of the disease and 1 is alive at the time of the report. Out of the remaining 8, six were alive at the time of the report and two dead for other causes. They all had been operated on (4) or locally irradiated with doses over 48 Gy. It should be noted that the original group included a high number of pts treated with smaller doses on the primary and lymph drainage (25-35 Gy). Only one of the 4 long survivors irradiated with higher doses had received chemotherapy, which is now considered insufficient (Chlorambucil only). Also with pts "cured" with the association of radiotherapy ancd chemotherapy, high doses seem important. Johnson (1985) report on 14 pts surviving for over 6 years out of 252 pts treated with chemotherapy only or associated with radiotherapy. Of these 14, 9, with limited disease, had been irradiated with at least 40 Gy (40-52 Gy). In Livingston's series (1984) 11 pts with limited disease - 10.7% of total number - are cured after combined treatment with 45 Gy total dose. Analysis of long survivals, however, are few and do not yield much information as to the factor we are interested in. The data referring to pts treated with radiotherapy only are even more scarce, for the limited use of this modality in recent years. A larger number of pts can be taken into account, although with the usual cautions, if

we analyse in retrospect data on 2-year survivors with limited disease, treated in different centres with radiotherapy only. Carr (1972) reports 2-year 11% survival in 27 pts treated with radiotherapy only and 45-50 Gy total doses. 13% of 33 pts with SCLC treated by Petrovich (1978) with radiotherapy only (50-60 Gy) survive after 2 years. 2-year survival is 5% in 121 pts, among those registered in the second MRC study, treated with radiotherapy only and a total dose of 30 Gy (Bleehen, 1981). Cox (1979) reported on 69 pts. 35 had been treated with local radiotherapy only -9 out of 35 (25%) presented "extended disease"-; 9   with local radiotherapy plus total body irradiation -4 out of 9 (45%) with "extended disease"-; 25 with local radiotherapy and chemotherapy -22 out of 25 (88%) with "extended disease"-. In the local radiotherapy only group relapses concentrated in the 16 pts who had been given total doses under 1600 ret (corresponding to about 50 Gy with conventional fractionation); 75% of these pts relapsed (12/16). Local control was, instead, excellent with doses above 1600 ret: 21% only (4/19) relapsed. Differences in local control according to dose were not evident in the two groups were a systemic form of treatment had been associated. However, the dose used in these two groups had been above 1600 ret in one case only. Moreover, the best local control obtainable with lower doses in the group treated with chemotherapy or total body irradiation might have been also due to the reduction in reseeding of the area of the primary starting from the peripheral sites of the disease, thanks to the systemic therapy used. In fact, 25% of the cases in the group treated with local radiotherapy only had "extended disease". In one of his more recent reports (Byhardt, 1982), Cox himself specifies that the necessary total dose, in the order of 60-65 Gy when radiotherapy only is used, should not be under 50 Gy, even when chemotherapy is associated. Huang (1985) has tried to correlate local control with total dose in 50 pts also treated with chemotherapy. Comparing the group treated with total doses between 996 and 1018 ret -3/6 pts with "extended disease"-with that treated with doses over 1543 ret -11/28 pts with "extended disease"-, 1 - year survival goes from 0 up to 21.4%, confirming what previously observed. Other reports suggest a relationship between an increase in total dose and local control of the disease in both the cases treated with radiotherapy only and in those given associated treatment. Choi (1976) present an actual dose-effect curve, with local control percentages from 60% in cases treated with 30 Gy (1133 ret) to 79% (40 Gy or 1361 ret) and 88% (48 Gy or 1518 ret). Despite the short follow up of these pts (4 months) there is a clear indication of the effects of the increased dose. White (1982) observed in 205 pts treated according to two different versions of a protocol of combined therapy by Southwest Oncology Group (SWOG) that those treated with a 45 Gy dose survived longer than those treated with 30 Gy, thanks to the better local control. A recent multicentric Canadian randomized study (Coy, 1986) evaluates the effects of two dose levels: 1087 ret (25 Gy in 10 fractions over two weeks) and 1415 ret (37,5 Gy in 15 fractions over three weeks) in association with chemoterapy, for the treatment of "limited disease" SCLC. The local progression-free survival was significantly higher in the high dose group.

TABLE 7   Incidence of Intrathoracic Relapses in Pts with "Limited Disease" Treated with Radiochemotherapy, According to the Equivalent Dose.

DOSE (RET)	RELAPSES (%)
1086	20/40 (50%)
1419	72/217 (33%)
1509	33/105 (31%)
1577	15/64 (23%)

Data processed from Perez (1984)

If we process the data collected by Perez (1984) about different groups of
pts treated with chemoradiotherapy in several centres we can see that local
control grows with the equivalent dose.
Finally, some autoptic studies have demonstrated that the disease disappears
more frequently from the irradiated volume, when higher doses are used. Besides
Rissanen's study (1968), Ajaikumar's series (1979) should be mentioned. 5 out
of the 30 cases considered by this Author did not present intrathoracic disease.
All of them had been treated with total doses of at least 45 Gy.
Radiotherapy with radical intent can be used alone and in association with
chemotherapy in limited disease. In both cases, the need to use high total
doses makes it necessary to limit the fractional dose and the volume to reduce
treatment-related complications. This need should not prevent carrying out
radiotherapy in the shortest possible time. In fact, if tumor repopulation
is an important factor in limiting cure possibilities, more rapid treatments
will increase cure rate.
A survey of the literature shows that the variation field of fractional dose
is very wide: 180, 200, 250, 280, 300, 320, 350 and 400 cGy 5 days a week or
even 3 or 4 times a week.
By using: a) Fowler's method (1983) to calculate the equivalent dose with fractionations different from the conventional one; b) the mean value from the
literature of the α/β ratio for the SCLC neoplastic tissue; c) the value
of the α/β ratio for lung tissue proposed by Tubiana (1986), we can calculate as an example that a 40 Gy total dose - with a 4 Gy fractional dose repeated
5 times a week - is equivalent, with conventional fractionation, to 44 Gy for
tumor tissue and 58 Gy for lung tissue. Hyperfractionation may be the answer
to the necessity to reduce the treatment overall time even with small fractional
doses. The feasibility of this technique also with lung tumors is demonstrated
by Saunders and Dische (1986 and 1987). It is now being experimented by several
groups for SCLC (Turrisi's is one of them).
Another controversial issue is the volume to be treated. The high percentage
of intrathoracic relapses in pts treated with chemotherapy only and an increase
in local control with increase in total doses when radiotherapy only or associated with chemotherapy is used seem to favour irradiation of the initial
tumor volume with adequate margins. Lymphatic drainage (mediastinum, hila,
supraclavear nodes) should be included. This ideal solution is opposed by:
a) the association of chemo- and radiotherapy increases the damage to healthy
tissues, particularly when the two are used simultaneously (Steel, 1983); b)
the necessary high total doses are not so well tolerated when on larger volumes.
Consequently greater damage would occur in those pts requiring larger volumes
for the greater local extension of the disease and whose prognosis is therefore
worse;this leads to a reduction in the therapeutic index of the treatment.
For this reason, some reports from the literature suggest irradiating the
residual tumor mass after chemotherapy when the latter is given first, inser-
ting a posterior shield to protect spinal cord and esophagus as from a certain
dose, reducing the dose given in association with chemotherapy to allow the
irradiation of larger volumes, not including the supraclavear nodes in the
treated volume with lower lobe primaries, not to be obliged to widen the volume
substantially. No operative agreement was reached at the Workshops in 1981
and 1984 of the International Association for the Study of Lung Cancer (Bleehen,
1983; Smith, 1985) as a consequence of this conflict. However, some of the
issues raised are no longer current. The greater availability of CT for treatment
planning diminishes the need for the cord and esophagus posterior shielding
owing to the fact that even the more complex treatment plans can be easily
and quickly worked out for the same purpose (Lichter, 1985). Efficient and
less toxic polichemotherapeutic schemes allow the simultaneous use of the two
modalities. In this case as well as with locally advanced forms treated with
radiotherapy only, one of the possible solutions is to use the "coning down" tech
nique. This way, the higher dose is given only to the tumor mass.

To conclude, the use of high total doses (50-60 Gy), of small fractions (180-200 cGy) and of the smallest possible volume improves the therapeutic index. Adherence to these standards implies a heavy workload and it is also demanding for the patients. This type of treatment should be used with radical intent. Total doses and optimal fractionation are naturally different when the treatment is done with symptomatic, palliative aim. The Authors too feel that pts with "extended disease" should not be aggressively treated. This opinion has been authoritatively confirmed by some of the participants at the Consensus Meeting held at St. Thomas in March 1986. Radiotherapy-chemotherapy routine association, therefore, does not seem to be indicated in these cases and most of the therapeutic protocols for "extended disease" does not envisage it. The exceptional cures in pts at this stage were almost always obtained with chemotherapy only (Byhardt, 1983; Einhorn, 1978; Maurer, 1980; Morstyn, 1984; Peschel, 1981). However, there is very little doubt that irradiation of symptomatic extrathoracic lesions is the shortest and simplest way to obtain remission of symptoms in the majority of cases. This is true, for example, for bone lesions, particularly frequent, or for those of the spinal cord, more frequently observed owing to the lenghtening of life span obtained with chemotherapy in recent years (Byhardt, 1982). Moreover, even if some Authors (Ochs, 1983) consider SCLC intrathoracic manifestations less responsive to radiotherapy after failure of chemotherapy, in these cases radiotherapy seems to offer better results, in terms of responses, than further "second line" chemotherapy (Morstyn 1984).
In all the above cases the choice for symptomatic radiotherapy is arrived at by trying to reduce the time necessary for the therapy and the treatment - induced complications in pts with short expectation of life. In this situation it is right to use smaller total doses and sometimes to resort to hypofractionation in order to reduce hospital stay or visits. Fractional dose should nevertheless be cautiosly increased in case of SVC syndrom.
Moreover, particular problems arise from the systemic use of radiotherapy. A relatively small number of studies has evaluated the effectiveness of total body irradiation (TBI) and sequential irradiation (SHI) of the upper and lower hemi body in SCLC.
This type of treatment has sometimes been associated with locoregional radiotherapy with different total doses, in pts with "limited" or "extended" disease. For both TBI and SHI different total doses and fractionations have been used. The frequency of even very severe collateral effects, mostly involving the lung, has prouved to be strictly dependent on these variables as could be gathered from previous studies on the lung tolerance to irradiation. TBI studies in SCLC have been carried out with fractionated treatment and low fractional and total doses, on the trace of what had already been experimented in lymphomas. There has not been, as foreseeable, a particularly high incidence of complications, but, notwithstanding the rather high complete remission rate in the cases treated also with radiotherapy on the primary, the disease-free interval was short and the mean survival time was not affected (Lichter, 1985). The interest has therefore been focused on SHI and upper hemibody irradiation (UHBI) generally done with single fractions and relatively high doses. A mild increase in the total dose over 8 Gy in single session may cause a marked increase in fatal complications. Fractionation may substantially contribute to reducing the incidence of radiation pneumonitis, for the same total dose. The clearly satisfying results obtained with UHBI and SHI when associated with local radiotherapy make these techniques competitive with chemotherapy in the treatment of pts with limited disease although the majority of Authors use them to "consolidate" chemotherapy results (Dawes, 1980; Eichorn, 1983; Payne, 1983; Powell, 1986; Salazar, 1980 and 1981; Urtasun, 1982). Even in the case of the prophylactic treatment of areas difficult to reach for drugs ("sanctuaries"), total dose and the most suitable modalities for its administration should be carefully chosen. Brain irradiation is the most difficult problem. Unlike the irradiation of the upper hemiabdomen the prophylactic irradiation of this area has

substantially reduced the number of relapses after chemotherapy . There is no proof, however, that prophylactic brain irradiation (PBI) can significantly prolong survival, except, perhaps, in the group of pts who achieved a CR (Lichter, 1985). A certain number of reports (Johnson, 1985; Lee, 1986) present data on the appearance of neurological deficits in pts treated with PBI and aggressive chemotherapy. Methotrexate (Lee, 1986) and Cisplatinum (Murray, 1986) are among the potentially neurotoxic drugs used in association with radiotherapy. Rather than reduce PBI total dose from 30 to 24 Gy as proposed by Lichter to decrease complications, it seems more sensible to keep the dose per fraction within 2 Gy, considering that nervous system has a quite low α/β ratio and also that relapses are more frequent with lower doses (Hoskin, 1986). Recent studies seem to demonstrate that the use of accelerated fractionation with fractional doses not higher than 2 Gy does not increase the toxicity of irradiation (D'Elia, 1986).

CONCLUSIONS

Considering the premises previously discussed, SCLC treatment results cannot be said to be less frustrating for the oncologist nowadays   than they were 10-15 years ago. A possibility of cure or at least of a significant extension of survival exist for those cases with "limited disease". Apart from pts with truly limited disease (T_{1-2} N_0 M_0) an increase in the percentage of long survivors is likely to depend on the optimal integration of local radiotherapy with currently available systemic treatment.   Even a small increase in the number of long survivors has great significance in a disease so rapidly and almost invariably fatal. One should therefore choose the "systemic" treatment which gives the best results with the least possible damage: even the reduction in the treatment - free life time brought about by certain protocols should be considered damage.

As regards radiotherapy, the most promising alternatives seem to be the use of hyper - or conventional fractionation for a total dose which must be as high as the one regarded as optimal for other lung malignancies (50-60 Gy). Besides a substantial workload and a rather complicated organization, hyperfractionation requires accurate monitoring as regards the frequently important acute reactions, of esophagus and bronchi, for example. The Authors therefore feel that the use of this type of fractionation should be limited, at present, to clinical protocols in large centers. Turrisi (1986 and in the Abstracts of this Congress) has obtained 92% of CR with 70% of relapse-free pts and a median 17 months follow-up - in pts with "limited disease" - with a hyperfractionation scheme started almost simultaneously (within 24 hours) with chemotherapy, firstly with Cisplatinum and Etoposide and going on in alternate cycles with "CAV" for a total of 6 cycles.

As regards systemic therapy, in fact, the two chemotherapy schemes whose effectiveness seems to have been fully demonstrated are those with Cyclophosfamide, Adriamycin and Vincristin ("CAV") suggested by Livingston (1978) and that with Cisplatinum and Etoposide ("PE") which seems to be an acceptable alternative to the former (Einhorn, 1987). The latter scheme is more easily integrated in a protocol of combined therapy for the absence of Adriamycin. The recent re-evaluation of the role of radiotherapy in SCLC has, among the other things, led to recognizing the importance of an early beginning of radiation therapy. This element as well as the prouven greater effectiveness of those protocols which use chemotherapy and radiotherapy simultaneously (Catane, 1981) have led to prefer the PE scheme in combined modality treatments for its lower toxicity in this setting (McCracken, 1986). The SWOG protocol described by McCracken and that of Turrisi share the use of limited fractional doses (150 and 180 cGy), the association of radiotherapy and PE and three-month "consolidation" chemotherapy. The total duration of treatment is therefore

about six months. It is short if compared with that of the many protocols which envisage "maintenance chemotherapy" but quite long if compared with the mean survival of these pts.
The possibility of substituting chemotherapy with SHI and UHBI as systemic treatments has not yet sufficiently been explored within "ad hoc" trials. Chemotherapy for SCLC has certainly increased the pts mean survival, but any substantial increase in long term cures has not yet been demonstrated. The data in the previous paragraphs and the evident decrease in intrathoracic relapses in pts with limited disease when locoregional radiotherapy is added to chemotherapy (Lichter, 1985 and Perez, 1986) demonstrate that radiotherapy is an essential component in the treatment of these pts. Moreover, there is sufficient clinical evidence to assume that SHI and UHBI are effective alternatives to chemotherapy as systemic treatments. Urtasun (1982) has treated a series of 30 pts with SHI and local radiotherapy, comparing the results, in a randomized fashion, with those obtained with chemotherapy instead of SHI. Although the two groups included pts with extended disease for whom SHI effectiveness is more debatable (Salazar, 1981), both the clinical response and survival rate were the same. Eichorn (1983) obtained similar results, although outside a randomized study. The integration of SHI (or UHBI) and chemotherapy is possible, both electively and using, "as needed", one of the two modalities when the other fails (Powell, 1986; Urtasun, 1983). Most of the Authors quoted here have not observed any increase in the toxicity of chemotherapy for the addiction of SHI. The elective combination of SHI and chemotherapy as systemic treatment seems however less logical than their alternative use. No substantial differences emerge from the comparison of the toxicities of the two modalities. However, the duration of gastroenteric symptoms and of haematological alterations has been obviously shorter in the cases treated with SHI.
In conclusion, we feel that radiotherapy has an important role in the treatment of SCLC, symptomatically and palliatively as well as when aiming at cure.
More extensive clinical investigation of hyperfractionation in the local radiotherapy of SCLC and of SHI as prophylaxis of the disease systemic manifestations is to be wished for, also in order to improve the quality of life, considering the present short mean survival.
To this end it is important to select accurately the pts who need aggressive treatment. It is therefore essential to report the results obtained also in terms of survival for over two years after treatment in pts staged according to the TNM system.

REFERENCES

Ajaikumar, B.S. and Barkley, H.T. (1979). The role of radiation therapy in the treatment of SCLC, Int. J. Radiation Oncology Biol. Phys., 5, 977-982.
Bleehen, N.M. (1981). Radiotherapy alone or with chemotherapy in the treatment of small-cell carcinoma of the lung: the results at 36 months, Br. J. Cancer, 44, 611-617.
Bleehen, N.M., Bunn, P.A., Cox, J.D., Dombernowsky, P., Fox, R.M., Host, H., Joss, R., White, J.E. and Wittes, R.E. (1983). Role of radiotherapy in small cell anaplastic carcinoma of the lung, Cancer Treat. Rep., 67, 11-19.
Breur, K. (1966). Growth rate and radiosensitivity of human tumors, Europ. J. Cancer, 2, 157-188.
Brigham, B.A., Bunn, P.A., Minna J.D., Cohen, M.H., Ihde, D.C. and Shackney S.E. (1978). Growth rates of small cell bronchogenic carcinomas, Cancer, 42, 2880-2886.

Byhardt, M.D., Cox, J.D., Holoye, P.Y. and Libnoch, J.A. (1982). The role of consolidation irradiation in combined modality therapy of small cell carcinoma of the lung, Int. J. Radiation Oncology, Biol. Phys., 8, 1271-1276.

Byhardt, R.W. and Cox, J.D. (1983). Is chest radiotherapy necessary in any or all patients with small cell lung cancer? Yes., Cancer Treat. Rep., 67, 209-215.

Byhardt, R.W., Hartz, A., Libnoch, J.A., Hansen, R. and Cox, J.D. (1986). Prognostic influence of TNM staging and LDH levels in small cell carcinoma of the lung (SCLC), Int. J. Radiation Oncology, Biol. Phys., 12, 771-777.

Carney, D.N., Mitchell, J.B. and Kinsella, J.J. (1983). In vitro radiation and chemotherapy sensitivity of established cell lines of human small cell lung cancer and its large cell morphological variants, Cancer Res., 43, 2806-2811.

Carr, D.T., Childs, D.S. and Lee, R.E. (1972). Radiotherapy plus 5-FU compared to radiotherapy alone for inoperable and unresectable bronchogenic carcinoma, Cancer, 29, 375-380.

Carr, D.T. and Mountain, C.F. (1983). Staging lung cancer, In M.J. Straus (Ed.) Lung cancer, Grune & Stratton, New York, Chap. 13, pp. 201-212.

Carter, D. and Eggleston, J.C. (1981). Small cell carcinoma, In Atlas of Tumor Pathology, Castle House Publication, second Series, Fascicle 17, pp. 95-113.

Cataldo, I., Bedini, A.V., Santoro, A., Bidoli, P. and Ravasi, G. (1987). In Program and abstracts of the International Conference on Small Cell Lung Cancer, Ravenna, p. 137.

Catane, R., Lichter, A. and Lee, Y.J. (1981). Small cell lung cancer: analysis of treatment factors contributing to prolonged survival, Cancer, 48, 1936-1943.

Chahinian, P. (1972). Relationship between tumor doubling time and anatomo-clinical features in 50 measurable pulmonary cancers, Chest, 61, 340-345.

Chai, C.H. and Carey, R.W. (1976). Small cell lung Cancer. Reappraisal of the current management, Cancer, 37, 2651-2657.

Cionini, L., Pacini, P., De Paola, E., Corrado, A., De Luca Cardillo, C., Mungai, V., Biti G.P. and Ponticelli, P. (1984). Respiratory function tests after mantle irradiation in patients with Hodgkin's disease, Acta Radiol. Oncology, 23, 401-410.

Cohen, M.H. and Matthews, M.J. (1978). Small cell bronchogenic carcinoma: a distinct clinico-pathologic entity, Semin. Oncol., 5, 234-243.

Cox, J.D., Byhardt, R., Komaki, R., Wilson, J.F., Libnoch, J.A. and Hansen, R. (1979). Interaction of thoracic irradiation and chemotherapy on local control and survival in small cell carcinoma of the lung, Cancer Treat. Rep., 63, 1251-1255.

Coy, P., Evans, W.K., Feld, R., Hodson, I., MacDonald, A.S., Osoba, D., Payne, D.G. and Pater, J.L. (1986). Canadian multicentre randomized trial comparing two dose levels of thoracic radiation given in combination with chemotherapy to patients with limited small cell lung cancer, Int. J. Radiation Oncology Biol. Phys., 12 (Sup. 1), 157.

Darves, P.J.D.K. (1980). Results of a pilot study of wide field radiotherapy in the treatment of oat cell carcinoma of the bronchus, Clin. Radiol., 31, 723-727.

Deacon, J., Peckham, M.J., Steel, G.G. (1984). The radioresponsiveness of human tumors and the initial slope of the cell survival curve, Radiotherapy and Oncology, 2, 317-323.

D'Elia, F., Bonucci, I., Biti, G.P., Pirtoli, L. (1986). Different fractiona-tion schedules in radiation treatment of cerebral metastases, Acta Radiol. Oncol., 25, 181-184.

Denekamp, J. (1983). Does physiological hypoxia matter in cancer therapy? In G.G. Steel, G.E. Adams and M.J. Peckham (Eds.), The biological basis of Radio-therapy, Elsevier, Amsterdam, Chap. 11, pp. 139-155.

Duchesne, G.M., Peacock, J.H.,   and Steel, G.G. (1986). The acute in vitro and in vivo radiosensitivity of human lung tumor lines, Radiotherapy and Oncology, 7, 353-361.

Eichorn, H.J., Hüttner, J., Dallüge, K.H. and Welker, K. (1983). Preliminary report on "one-time" and high dose irradiation of the upper and lower half-body in patients with small cell lung cancer, Int. J. Radiation Oncology Biol. Phys., 9, 1459-1465.

Einhorn, L.H., Bond, W.H. and Hornback, H. (1978). Long term results in combined modality treatment of small cell carcinoma of the lung, Semin. Oncol., 5, 309-313.

Einhorn, L.H. (1986). Cisplatin plus UP-16 in small-cell lung cancer, Semin. Oncol. 13, (Sup. 3), 3-4.

Fertil., B., Malaise, E.P. (1981). Inherent radiosensitivity as a basic concept for human tumor radiotherapy, Int.J.Radiation Oncology, Biol. Phys., 7, 621-629.

Fowler, J.F. (1983). Fractionation and therapeutic gain. In G.G. Steel, G.E. Adams, M.J. Peckham (Eds). The biological basis of radiotherapy, Elsevier, Amsterdam, Chap. 14, pp. 181-194.

Fowler, J.F. (1986). Potential for increasing differential response between tumors and normal tissues: can proliferation rate be used? Int. J. Radiation Oncology Biol. Phys., 12, 641-645.

Fox, W. and Scadding J.G. (1973). Medical Research Council comparative trial of surgery and radiotherapy for primary treatment of small-celled or oat-celled carcinoma of the bronchus, Lancet, 2, 63-65.

George, T.K., Fitzgerald, D., Brown, B.S., Chuang, C., Asbury R.F., and Boros, L. (1986). Long term survival in limited-stage small cell lung cancer, Cancer, 58, 1193-1198.

Goodwin, G. and Baylin, S.B. (1982). Relationships between neuroendocrine differentiation and sensitivity to γ-radiation in culture line OH-1 of human small cell lung carcinoma, Cancer Res., 42, 1361-1367.

Hirsch, F.R., Osterlind, K. and Hansen, H.H. (1983). The prognostic significance of histopathologic subtyping of small cell carcinoma of the lung according to the classification of the World Health Association, Cancer, 52, 2144-2150.

Hoskin, P.J., Yarnold, J.R., Smith, I.E. and Ford, H.T. (1986). CNS relapse despite prophylactic cranial irradiation (PCI) in small cell lung cancer (SCLC), Int. J. Radiation Oncology Biol. Phys., 12, 2025-2028.

Huang H.N. (1985). Clinical analysis of combination chemotherapy plus radiation therapy for small cell undifferentiated carcinoma of the lung, Clinical Oncology, 12, 216-219.

Ihde, D.C. and Hansen H.H. (1981). Staging procedures and prognostic factors in small cell carcinoma of the lung. In F.A. Greco and P.A. Bumm (Eds). Small cell lung Cancer, Grune & Stratton, New York, Chap. 11, pp. 261-283.

Johnson, B.E., Ihde, D.C., Bunn, P.A., Becker, B., Walsh, T., Weinstein, Z.R., Matthews, M.J., Whang-Peng, J., Makuch, R.W., Johnston-Early, A., Lichter, A.S., Carney, D.N., Cohen, M.H., Glatstein, E. and Minna, J. D. (1985). Patients with small-cell lung cancer treated with combination chemotherapy with or without irradiation, Am. Intern. Med., 103, 403-439.

Kallman, R.F. and Dorie, M.J. (1986). Tumor oxygenation and reoxygenation during radiation therapy: their importance in predicting tumor response, Int. J. Radiation Oncology Biol. Phys., 12, 681-685.

Kerr, K.M. and Lamb, D. (1984). Actual growth rate and tumor cell proliferation in human pulmonary neoplasms, Br. J. Cancer, 50, 343-349.

Laing, A.H. and Berry, R.J. (1975). Treatment of small-cell carcinoma of bronchus, Lancet, 1, 129-132.

Lee, J.S., Umsawasdi, T., Lee, Y.Y., Barkley, H.T., Murphy, W.K., Welch, S. and Valdivieso, M. (1986). Neurotoxicity in long-term survivors of small cell lung cancer, Int. J. Radiation Oncology Biol. Phys., 12, 313-321.

Libshitz, H.I., Brosof, A.B., Southard, M.E. (1973). Radiographic appearance of the chest following extended field radiation therapy for Hodgkin's disease, Cancer, 32, 206-215.

Lichter, A.S., Bunn, P.A., Ihde, D.C., Cohen, M.H., Makuch, R.W., Carney, D.N.,

Johnston-Early, A., Minna, J.D. and Glatstein, E. (1985). The role of radiation therapy in the treatment of small cell lung cancer, Cancer, 55, 2163-2175.

Livingston, R.B., Moore, T.N., Heilbrun, M.D. (1978). Small cell carcinoma of the lung combined chemotherapy and radiation, Am. Int. Med., 88, 194-199.

Livingston, R.B., Stephens, R.L., Bonnett, J., Grozca, P.N. and Lehane, D.E. (1984). Long-term survival and toxicity in small cell lung cancer, Am. J. Med., 77, 415-417.

Malaise, E.P., Charbit, A. and Tubiana, N. (1972). Change in volume of irradiated metastases. Investigation of repair of sublethal damage and tumor repopulation, Br. J. Cancer, 26, 43-52.

Malaise, E.P., Chavandra, N. and Tubiana, M. (1973). The relationship between growth rate, labelling index and histological type of human solid tumors, Eur. J. Cancer, 9, 305-312.

Malaise, E.P., Fertil, B., Chavandra, N. and Guichard, M. (1986). Distribution of radiation sensitivities for human tumor cells of specific histological types, Int. J. Radiation Oncology Biol. Phys., 12, 617-624.

Matthews, M.J., Gazdar,A.F. (1981). Pathology of small cell carcinoma of the lung and its subtypes. A clinico-pathological correlation. In R.B. Livingston (Ed) Lung cancer 1, Martinus Nijhoff Publishers, The Hagne, Chap. 10, pp. 283-306.

Maurer, L.H., Tulloh, M., Weiss, R.B., Blom. J., Leone, L., Glidewell, O. and Pajak, T.F. (1980). A randomized combined modality trial in small cell carcinoma of the lung, Cancer, 45, 30-39.

Mauro, F., Teodori, L., Schumann, J. and Göhde, W. (1986). Flow cytometry as a tool for the prognostic assessment of human neoplasia, Int. J. Radiation Oncology Biol. Phys., 12, 625-636.

McCracken, J., Janaki, L., Taylor, S., Shankar Giri, P.G., Weiss, G.B., Gordon, W., Vance, R.B. and Crowley, J. (1986). Concurrent chemotherapy and radiotherapy for limited small-cell carcinoma of the lung: a southwest oncology group study, Sem. Oncol., 3 (Sup. 3), 31-36.

Meyer, J.A. (1973). Growth rate VS prognosis in resected primary bronchogenic carcinoma, Cancer, 31, 1468-1472.

Morstin, G., Ihde, D.C., Lichter, A.S., Bunn, P.A., Carney, D.N., Glatstein, E. and Minna, J. (1984). Small cell lung cancer 1973-1983: early progress and recent obstacles, Int. J. Radiation Oncology Biol. Phys., 10, 515-539.

Murray, N. (1986). St. Thomas Consensus on the treatment of small-cell lung cancer, Sem. Oncol., 13 (Sup. 3), 83-86.

Ochs, J.J., tester, W.J., Cohen, M.H., Lichter, A.S., Ihde, D.C. (1983). "Salvage" radiation therapy for intrathoracic small cell carcinoma of the lung progressing on combination chemotherapy, Cancer Treat. Rep., 67, 1123-1126.

Olsson, L., Sorensen, H.R. and Behnke, O. (1984). Intratumoral phenotypic diversity of cloned human lung tumor cell lines and consequences for analyses with monoclonal antibodies, Cancer, 54, 1757-1766.

Payne, D.G., Yeoh, L., Feld, R., Pringle, J.F., Evans, W.K., Herman, J.G. and Quirt, I.C. (1983). Upper half body irradiation (UHBI) for extensive small cell carcinoma of the lung, Int. J. Radiation Oncology Biol. Phys., 9, 1571-1574.

Perez, C.A., Einhorn, L., Oldham, R.K., Greco, F.A., Cohen, H.J., Silberman, H., Krauss, S., Hornback, N., Comas, F., Omura, G., Salter, M., Keller, J. W., McLaren, J., Kellermeyer, R., Storaasli, J., Birch, R. and Dandy M. (1984). Randomized trial of radiotherapy to the thorax in limited small-cell carcinoma of the lung treated with multi-agent chemotherapy and elective brain irradiation: a preliminary report, J. Clin. Oncol., 2, 1200-1208.

Perez, C., Bauer, M., Edelstein, S., Gillespie, B.W. and Birch, R. (1986). Impact of tumor control on survival in carcinoma of the lung treated with irradiation, Int. J. Radiation Oncology Biol. Phys., 12, 539-547.

Peschel, R.E., Kapp, D.S., Carter, D. and Knowlton, A. (1981). Long term survivors with small cell carcinoma of the lung, Int. J. Radiation Oncology Biol. Pys., 7, 1545-1548.

Peters, L.J., Withers, H.R., Thames, H.D. and Fletcher, G. (1982). Keynote address the problem: tumor radioresistance in clinical radiotherapy, Int. J. Radiation Oncology Biol. Phys., 8, 101-108.

Peters, L.J., Brock, W.A., Johnson, T., Meyn, R.E., Tofilon, P.J. and Milas, L. (1986). Potential methods for predicting tumor radiocurability, Int. J. Radiation Oncology, Biol. Phys., 12, 459-467.

Petrovich, Z., Ohanian, M., and Cox, J. (1978). Clinical research on the treatment of locally advanced lung cancer, Cancer, 42, 1129-1134.

Powell, B., Jackson, D.V., Scarantino, C.W., Pope, E.K., Douglas Case, L., Choplin, R., Richards, F., Muss, H.B., Craig, J.B., Cruz, J.M., Zekan, P.J., McMahan, R.A., White, D.R., Stuart, J.J., Woodruff, R.D., Spurr, C.L., Capizzi, R.L. (1986). Sequential hemibody irradiation integrated into a chemotherapy - local radiotherapy program for limited disease small cell lung cancer, Int. J. Radiation Oncology, Biol. Phys., 12, 1951-1956.

Raber, M., Barlogie, B., Farquhar, D. (1980). Determination of ploidy abnormality and cell cycle time distribution in human lung cancer using DNA flow cytometry, Proceedings of the American Association for Cancer Research, 21, 40.

Rissanen, P.M., Tikka, U. and Holsti, L.R. (1968). Autopsy findings in lung cancer treated with megavoltage radiotherapy, Acta Radiol. Ther. Phys. Biol. 7, 433-442.

Rubin, P., Casarett, G.W. (1972). A directory for clinical radiation pathology: the tolerance dose, Front. Radiat. Ther. Oncol., 6, 345-355.

Russo, A., Kinsella, T. (1985). Determinants of radiosensitivity, Semin. Oncol., 12, 332-349.

Salazar, O.M., Creech, R.H., Rubin, P., Bennett, J.M., Mason, B.A., Young, J.J., Scarantino, C.W., Catalano, R.B. (1980). Half-body and local chest irradiation as consolidation following response to standard induction chemotherapy for disseminated small cell lung cancer, Int. J. Radiation Oncology, Biol. Phys., 6, 1093-1102.

Salazar, O.M., Zagars, G. (1981). Radiation therapy-new approaches. In R.B. livingston (Ed) Lung Cancer 1, Martinus Nijhoff Publishers, The Hagne, Chap. 9, pp. 209-281.

Saunders, M.I. and Dische S. (1986). Radiotherapy employing three fractions in each day over a continuous period of 12 days, Br. J. Radiol., 59, 523-525.

Saunders, M.I. and Dische, S. (1987). Radiotherapy employing 3 fractions each day over a continuous period of 12 days, Abstracts 6th ESTRO Annual Meeting, p. 184.

Shackney, S.E., McCormack, G.W. and Cuchural, G. (1978). Growth rate patterns of human solid tumors and their relation to response to therapy: an analytic review, Ann. Intern. Med., 89: 107-121.

Silvestrini R., Daidone, M.G. and Gasparini, G. (1985). Cell kinetics as a prognostic marker in node-negative breast cancer, Cancer, 56, 1982-1987.

Smith, J.F., Hansen, H.H. (1985). Current status of reserach into small cell carcinoma of the lung: summary of the 2nd Workshop of The International Association for the study of lung cancer (IASLC), Eur. J. Cancer Clin, Oncol., 21, 1295-1298.

Steel, G.G. (1983). The combination of radiotherapy and chemotherapy. In G.G. Steel, G.E. Adams, M.J. Peckham (Eds), The biological basis of radiotherapy, Elsevier, Amsterdam, Chap. 18, pp. 239-248.

Straus, M.J. (1974). The growth characteristics of lung cancer and its application to treatment design, Semin. Oncol., 1, 167-174.

Straus, M.J., Moran, R.E., Shackney, S.E. (1983). Growth characteristics of lung cancer. In M.J. Straus (Ed.) Lung cancer, Grune & Stratton, New York,

Chap. 2, pp. 21-35.

Thames, H.D. and Suit, H.D. (1986). Tumor radioresponsiveness versus fractionation sensitivity, Int. J. Radiation Oncology Biol. Phys., 12, 687-691.

Tubiana, M. and Malaise, E. (1977). Combination of radiotherapy and chemotherapy:
implications of cell kinetics. In F. Muggia and M. Rozencweig (Eds.) Lung
cancer, Raven Press, New York.

Tubiana, M. (1983). The causes of clinical radioresistance. In G.G. Steel,
G.E. Adams and M.J. Peckham (Eds.), The Biological basis of radiotherapy,
Elsevier, Amsterdam, Chap. 2, pp. 13-33.

Tubiana, M., Pejovic, M.H., Chavandra, G., Contesso, G. and Malaise, E.P.
(1984). The long term prognostic significance of the thymidine labelling
index in breast cancer, Int. J. Cancer, 33, 441-445.

Tubiana, M., Dutreix, J. and Wambersie, A. (1986). Radiobiologie, Hermann,
Paris, Chap. V, pp. 135-136.

Turrisi, A.T., Glover, D.J. (1986). The penn regimen (concurrent twice-daily
radiotherapy and platinum-etoposide) in limited small cell lung cancer,
Int. J. Radiation Oncology Biol. Phys., 12 (Sup. 1), 158.

Urtasum, R.C. Belch, A.R., Mckinnon, S., Higgins, E., Saunders, W. and Feld-
stein, M. (1982). Small cell lung cancer: initial treatment with sequential
hemi-body irradiation VS 3-drug systemic chemotherapy, Br. J. Cancer, 46,
228-235.

Vindelow, L.L., Hansen, H.H., Christensen, I.J., Spnag-Thomsen, M., Hirsch,
F.R., Hansen, M. and Nissen, N.I., Clonal heterogeneity of small-cell ana-
plastic carcinoma of the lung demonstrated by flow-cytometric DNA analysis,
Cancer Res., 40, 4295-4300.

Weichselbaum, R.R. (1986). Radioresistant and repair proficient cells may determine radiocurability in human tumors, Int. J. Radiation Oncology Biol. Phys.,
12, 637-639.

Whang-Peng, J., Kao-Shang, C.S., Lee, E.C., Bum, P.A., Carney, D.N., Gazdar,
A.F. and Minna, J.D. (1982). Specific chromosome defect associated with human
small-cell lung cancer: deletion 3 p (14-23), Science, 215, 181-182.

White J.E., Chen, T., McCracken, J., Kennedy, P., Seydel, H.G., Hartman, G.,
Mira, J., Khan, M., Durrance, F.Y., Skinner, O. (1982). The influence of
radiation therapy quality control on survival, response and sites of relapse
in oat cell carcinoma of the lung, Cancer, 50, 1084-1090.

Antiemetic Treatment and Parenteral Nutrition as Supports of Intensive Treatments of Small Cell Lung Cancer (SCLC)

A. Ardizzoni, V. Fusco, S. Chiara,
M. Gulisano, P. Pronzato and R. Rosso

Istituto Nazionale per la Ricerca sul Cancro,
V. le Benedetto XV, 10 – 16132 Genova, Italy

ABSTRACT

The recent results of supportive therapy in SCLC patients treated with intensive chemo-radiotherapic programs are hereby reported. Randomized trials concerning the use of PN during induction therapy are analized. To date there seems to be no clear advantage in terms of survival and chemotherapy related toxicities for pts receiving PN. Considering the considerable costs and related toxicities, the widespread use of PN in the corrent management of SCLC pts. is therefore not warranted.
On the contrary notable improvements in the control of high-dose -cisplatin induced nausea and vomiting have been reached. More than 80% complete emetic protection (0 emetic episodes) has been obtained with the use of high-dose meto-clopramide and steroids.
No definitive data concerning antiemetic management of non-cisplatin containing chemotherapy are currently available. In our experience steroids are effective and safe drugs suitable for use in this setting.

INTRODUCTION

Major advances in the treatment of SCLC have been obtained in the last two decades: 90% of patients are reported to be achieved objective response with disease free survival of 10-20% at 3 or more years. These results have been achieved with the aggressive use of multidrug chemotherapy and combination treatment, at the cost of a parallel increase in treatment related toxicities. As a consequence, currently, attention has been focused to overcome important side effects in order to allow the correct completion of intensive therapeutic programs.

ANTIEMETIC TREATMENT

Nausea and vomiting are frequent and serious toxicities in patients receiving cancer chemotherapy. The inability to control severe emesis may lead to post-ponement of therapy or to reduction of active drug doses; on the other hand it may be responsible for patients non-compliance and refusal of potentially curative therapy (Lazlo, 1983). Additional complications produced by prolonged nausea and vomiting may include severe dehydration, electrolyte imbalance, malnutrition and rarely esophageal tears and pathologic fractures.

Since no antiemetic trial has been conducted in patients receiving chemotherapy
for SCLC, data for antiemetic treatment in this disease are mainly infered from
studies concerning management of cisplatin-induced nausea and vomiting.
Historically these toxicities have been managed primarly with single-agent
therapy. Active antiemetic drugs tested in randomized studies include metoclopramide, steroids, cannabinoids and phenothiazines (Markmann 1984, Sallan 1980);
best results have been obtained with either high-dose metoclopramide or dexameta
sone (Gralla, 1984; Cassileth, 1983). However no currently available single agent
has been demonstrated to be completely effective. Combination regimens have
therefore become increasingly popular. The rationale for combining antiemetics
is based on the fact that chemotherapy-induced emesis is probably mediated
through multiple sites and different neurotrasmitters (Perontka, 1982).
Therefore antiemetics would be chosen according to the following principle:
proven single-agent efficacy, different mechanism and site of action, non
additive toxicities.
A major contribution in improving the control of CDDP-induced emesis comes from
the Memorial Sloan Kettering Cancer Center where studies, that included a large
population of lung cancer patients, demonstrated the effectiveness of high-dose
metoclopramide   (2 mg/kg for 5 doses).

Gralla et al. undertook a series of consecutive trials in order to investigate
optimal dosage and schedule of metoclopramide alone and to study the efficacy
of combination treatment including metoclopramide, dexamethasone and diphenhydra
mine. Dexamethasone was selected because of its proven efficacy, and lack of
substantial side effects in comparison to metoclopramide. Diphenhydramine is a
useful adjunct which prevents acute dystonic reactions that occur in about 8-30%
of patients treated with metoclopramide. Results of trials demonstrated that
similar antiemetic efficacy could be achieved with a lower total dose of metoclopramide and fewer administration (3 mg/kg for 2 doses instead of 2 mg/kg for
5 doses). The combination of metoclopramide (3 mg/kg for 2 doses) plus dexametha
sone (20 mg 30 min before CDDP) plus diphenhydramine (50 mg 30 min before CDDP)
was found to produce complete control of emesis in 81% of patients with no
distonic reactions and generally decreased incidence of treatment induced side
effects (Kris, 1985).
Among the newer agents identified, lorazepam has proved to be a useful drug that
may improve the effectiveness of combination antiemetic regimens. We treated out
patients receiving chemotherapeutic agents with moderate to severe emetogenic
potential and experiencing refractory emesis, with lorazepam 1.25 mg/kg IV 30
min. before therapy. The majority of patients (84%) demonstrated an increased
tolerance to chemotherapy, in spite of the modest objective improvement of emesis:
amnesia, experimented by 47% of patients appeared to be the most probable cause
of improved patients acceptance (Campora, 1986). Other authors reported that lora
zepam appeared to decrease anxiety caused by chemotherapy and that it reduced the
incidence of neurological side effects induced by metoclopramide (Friedlander,
1983; Kris, 1985).
In order to ensure antiemetic protection in patients receiving chemotherapy
courses and to prevent anticipatory nausea and vomiting, we administered the
following combination to patients receiving CDDP containing regimens (CDDP= 50-
120 mg/m^2).
Antiemetic treatment consisted of metoclopramide 1 mg/kg Iv plus methylprednisolo
ne 40 mg Iv plus orphenadrine 40 mg IM and lorazepam 1.25 mg/kg IV, prior to
chemotherapy and repeated after 6 and 12 hours. Preliminary results demonstrated
the feasibility and effectiveness of the combination regimen: complete and major

antiemetic protection (0-2 emetic episodes) occured in 84% of patients while
adverse effects where minimal and consisted chiefly in mild sedation and sleepi-
ness (81%). Fourty-seven % of patients didn't remember receiving chemotherapy.
Data on antiemetic protection in subsequent chemotherapy courses are not yet
available.
Effective combination chemotherapies widely used in SCLC patients include CAV
(cyclophosphamide+adriamycin+vincristine) or CMC regimen (cyclophosphamide+metho-
trexate+CCNU). To date the antiemetic approach to non-CDDP containing therapies
is not well defined. The studies available suggest that phenothiazines, butyrophe
nones and moderate-dose metoclopramide are effective in controlling nausea and
vomiting induced by mild to moderately emetogenic agents (Moertel 1963, Strum 1982
The single-agent activity and minimal incidence of side effects made steroids
excellent candidates for administration both in outpatients basis and in
combination regimens.
In a randomized trial performed in our institute the antiemetic efficacy of me-
thylpredinsolone (375 mg divided in 3 doses) was compared to metoclopramide (1
mg/kg administered in 3 doses). Patients receiving the steroid experienced
significantly less nausea and vomiting (p>0.00005) : complete antiemetic
protection (0 ematic episodes) was observed in 58% of patients receiving mathyl-
prednisolone as compared with 20% of patients treated with metoclopramide (Campora, 1985).
A subsequent study confirmed the significant antiemetic activity of methylpredni
solone in patients treated with non-cisplatin chemotherapy ; in addition protection
was reproducible in patients receiving multiple chemotherapy courses and a lower
(120 mg) steroid dose was found to be equally effective (Chiara, in press). In
our experiences steroids are recomendable antiemetic drugs suitable for use in
outpatients receiving moderately emetogenic therapy. Even so the control of
vomiting is not complete in all patients and we are investigating the usefulness
of combination regimen which includes methylprednisolone, 120 mg., and lorazepam,
a drug with amnesic and anxiolitic properties.
Although additional work is necessary in the area of basic neuropharmacology and
the problem of anticipatory, delayed or persistent emesis is largely unexplored,
in the last year considerable progress has been made in the treatment of chemotherapy-induced nausea and vomiting. To date several classes of drugs have a
precise role in the antiemetic armamentarium and randomized studies can be
appropriately designed. However evaluation of results in antiemetic trials is
often influenced by the presence of confounding factors: use of chemotherapy
agents with different emetogenic potential, inclusion of patients previously
exposed to cancer chemotherapy, difference in P.S., stage and type of neoplastic
disease. Furthermore standardization of parameters such as evaluation criteria
and definition of response is imperative to make antiemetic trials comparable.
Only by setting stringent inclusion and evaluation criteria in future trials can
allow us to define the antiemetic treatment specific for the various commonly
used chemotherapy regimens.

PARENTERAL NUTRITION

Weight loss and malnutrition are frequently associated with cancer as a
consequence of either tumor-treatment or disease itself. In many neoplasms,
including SCLC, the presence of significant weight loss at diagnosis is
associated with a poor prognosis (Osterlind, 1982).Therefore, being actually
possible to give nutrition intravenously it would seem logical to provide this
supportive treatment with the aim of improve prognosis.

Theoretical advantage of PN should be:
1) reversal of paramethers of malnutrition
2) improvement of response rate and survival
3) reduction of treatment-related toxicity.
The issue of effects of PN on patients nutritional prophile has been focused in
studies carried out by Canadian investigators. Evans et al. found that PN led to
a significant increase in mean caloric intake and weight compared to controls
($p < 0.0001$); furthermore triceps skinfold thickness was mainteined and arm muscle
circumference was increased (Evans, 1985). The same group of investigators found,
in patients with SCLC, that PN resulted in a significant positive net energy
balance, but during the follow-up, was associated with prolonged anorexia and
negative energy balance regardless of disease outcome.
These small positive effects of PN on nutritional paramethers are counter balanced
by the high cost of the procedure and its toxicity. In 1981 the daily cost of PN
including only the fluid, the equipment to deliver it, and the lab tests to
monitor the nutritional therapy, had been extimated to be $ 200 (Russel, 1984).
Concerning toxicity Weiner (1985) in a randomized trial in SLCL patients, reported
40% fluid overload, 9% congestive heart failure, 24% catheter related problems,
46% infection. The issue of effects of PN get further complicated by the
demonstration in animals that it produces a significant increase in s-phase tumor
cells (Valdivieso, 1987). This fenomenon can translate either in a negative
effect accelerating tumor growth or in a positive one, increasing the drug-
sensitivity of the tumor.
Thus it is evident for these considerations that a clear indication for PN use in
SCLC patients would come from clinical randomized trial looking at response rate,
survival and treatment related toxicity.
Three of such trials have been published in letterature (Valdivieso 1987; Weiner
1985, Serrou 1982).
The study by M. Valdivieso (1987) included 65 previously untreated SCLC patients
randomized to receive or not to receive PN during their first two of three
courses of intensive induction chemotherapy.
R.S. Weiner (1985) reported their results in 119 SCLC patients randomized to
receive self-regulated oral diet or PN during the first 30 days of induction
chemotherapy (Serrou, 1982; Koretz, 1984).
The third randomized trial by Serrou (1982) included 39 SCLC patients receiving
induction chemotherapy with adriamycin, vincristine, VP16 and cyclophosphamide.
None of these studies was able to demonstrate any difference in response rate
and survival between PN and control arm. Neither advantage was seen in the group
of patients who had >5% pretreatment weight loss, low caloric intake, decreased
serum albumine or reduced total iron-binding capacity in the trial by G.H. Cla-
nan (1985).
It was hoped that administration of PN during induction chemotherapy, was able
to reduce chemotherapy-related toxicity in order to allow that full dose therapy
are given without major problems.
Valdivieso (1982) found no significant differences in myelosuppressive toxicity;
there were more documented infections and more febrile episodes in the PN arm
without statistically significance; the percent of hospital days spent with mu-
cositis or vomiting was significantly higher in the PN group.
Similarly Weiner (1985) found that PN did not ameliorate chemotherapy induced
toxicity; patients receiving PN had higher granulocyte counts on day 14 and 21
of the first cycle of chemotherapy likely caused by fever and infection associated
with PN rather than any nutritional effect on granulopoiesis.

Likewise in the study by Serrou (1982) there was no difference in gastrointestinal and hematological toxicity (Solassol, 1979).
These results on PN in SCLC patients are in line with those obtained in patients
with different neoplasm (Szeluga, 1987). Only one paper demonstred a statistically significant improved survival associated with the use of PN, in terminal
cancer patients (Brennan, 1981).
We therefore conclude with R.L. Koretz (1984) that there is "non significant
evidence developed to date that PN has a demonstrable positive effect" and that
".... it is unreasonable to encourage the widespread use of PN in
oncology".
New treatment modalities becoming more common such as high-dosetherapy with bone
marrow transplantation or the concurrent administration of radiation and chemotherapy may possibly gain benefit from PN. Only one randomized trial has been published dealing with nutritional support of bone marrow transplant recipients with
primarly hematological neoplasms that demonstrated no differences in the rate of
hematopoietic recovery or survival between PN and individualized central feeding
(Torosian, 1984).
However, further experience in this special field is needed before any final
conclusion can be drown.

REFERENCES

Brennan, M.F. (1981). Total parenteral nutrition in the cancer patients. N. Engl.
J. Med, 305, 375-382.
Campora, E., Chiara, S., Bruzzi, P., Scarsi, P., Rosso, R. (1985). The antiemetic
efficacy of methylprednisolone compared with metoclopramide in outpatients receiving adjuvant CMF chemotherapy for breast cancer: a randomized trial. Tumori, 71,
459-462.
Campora, E., Sertoli, M.R., Chiara, S. (1986). Improved tolerance to chemotherapy
with lorazepam in outpatients with refractory nausea and vomiting. Farmaci e Tera-
pia, 2, 115-117.
Cassileth, P.A., Lusk, E.J., Torri, S. (1983). Antiemetic efficacy of dexamethaso
ne therapy in patients receiving cancer chemotherapy. Arch Intern Med., 143, 1347-
1349.
Chiara, S., Campora, E., Lionetto, R., Bruzzi, P., Rosso, R.(in press). Methylpred
nisolone for the control of CMF-induced emesis. Am. J. Clin. Oncol.
Clamon, G.H., Feld, R., Evans, W.K., Weiner, R.S., Moran, E.M., Blum, R.H., Kramer,
B.S., Makuch, R.W., Hoffman, F.A., DeWys, W.D.(1985). Effect of adjuvant central
Iv hyperalimentation on the survival and response to treatment of patients with
small cell lung caner: a randomized trial. Cancer Treat. Rep., 69, 167-177.
Evans, W.K., Makuch, R., Clamon, G.H., Feld, R., Weiner, R.S., Moran, E., Blum, R.,
Sheperd, F.A., Jeejeebhoy, K.N., DeWys, W.D. (1985). Limited impact of total paren
teral nutrition on nutritional status during treatment for small cell lung cancer.
Cancer Res., 45, 3347-3353.
Friedlander, H.L., Sims, K., Kearsley, J.H. (1983). Impairment of recall improves
tolerance of cytotoxic chemotherapy. Lancet, 2, 686.
Gralla, R.J. (1981). High dose metoclopramide: effective antiemetic against ci-
splatin in randomized trials vc placebo and prochlorperazine. Proc. AACR/ASCO, 22,
420.
Gralla, R.J., Tyson, L.B., Bordin, L.A., Clark, R.A., Kelser, D.P., Kris, M.G.,
Kalman, L.B., Groshen, S. (1984). Antiemetic therapy: a review of recent studies
and report of a random assignment trial comparing metoclopramide with delta-9

tetrohydrocarrabinol. Cancer treat. Rep., 68, 163-172.

Kris, M.G., Gralla, R.J., Tyson, L.B., Clark, R.A., Kelsen, D.P., Reilly, L.K., Groshen, S., Bosl, G.J., Kalman, L.A. (1985). Improved control of cisplatin - induced emesis with hig-dose metoclopramide and with combination of metoclopramide, dexamethasone and diphenhydramine. Cancer, 55, 527-534.

Kris, M.G., Gralla, R.J., Clark, R.A., Tyson, L.B., Fiore, J.J., Kelsen, D.P., Groshen, S. (1985). Consecutive dose-finding trials adding lorazepam to the combination of metoclopramide plus dexamethasone: improved subjective effectiveness over the combination of diphenhydramine plus metoclopramide plus dexamethasone. Cancer Rep., 69, 1257-1262.

Koretz, R.L. (1984). Parenteral nutrition: is it oncologically logical? Clin. Oncol., 2, 534-538.

Lazlo, J. Emesis as limiting toxicity in cancer chemotherapy. In J. Lazlo, Williams and Wilkins (Ed.). Antiemetics and cancer chemotherapy, Baltimore, p.2, 1983.

Markmann, M., Sheidler, V., Ettinger, D.S., (1984). Antiemetic efficacy of dexamethasone. Randomized double blind, crossover study with chlorperazine in patients receiving cancer therapy. N. Engl. J. Med., 311, 549-552.

Moertel, G.C., Reitemeier, R.J., Gage, R.P. (1963). A controlled clinical evaluation of antiemetic drugs. Jama, 186, 116-118.

Osterlind, K. (1982). Prognostic factors in patients with small cell lung cancer. In Proceedings of the III Conference on lung cancer. Tokyo May 17-20, p. 1(1982).

Peroutka, S.J., Snyder, S.H. (1982). Antiemetics: neurotrasmitter receptor binding predicts therapeutic actions. Lancet, 1, 658-660.

Russel, D.McR., Shike, M., Marliss, E.B., Detsky, A.S., Shepherd, F.A., Feld, R., Evans, W.K., Jeejeebhoy, K.N. (1984). Effects of total parenteral nutrition and chemotherapy on the metabolic derangements in small cell lung cancer. Cancer Res. 44, 1706-1711.

Sallan, S.E., Cronin, C., Zalen, M. (1980). Antiemetics in patients receiving chemotherapy for cancer: a randomized comparison of delta-9-tetrahydrocannabinol and prochlorperazine. N. Engl. J. Med., 302, 135-138.

Serrou, B., Cupissol, D., Plagne, R., Boutin, R. Chollet, P., Carcassonne, Y., Michel, F.B. (1982). Follow-up of a randomized trial for oat cell carcinoma evaluating the efficacy of peripheral intravenous nutrition (PIVN) as adjunct treatment. Recent Results Cancer Res., 80, 246-253.

Solassol, C. (1979). Total parenteral nutrition with complete nutritive mixtures: an artificial gut in cancer patients. Nutr. Cancer, 1, 13-18.

Strum, S.B., Mc. Dermed, J.E., Pileggi, J., Riech, L.P., Whitaker, H.(1984). Intravenous metoclopramide: prevention of chemotherapy-induced nausea and vomiting. Cancer, 83, 1432-1439.

Szeluga, D.J., Stuart, R.K., Brookmeyer, R., Utermohlen, V., Santos, G.W. (1987). Nutritional support of bone marrow transplant recipients: a prospective, randomized clinical trial comparing total parenteral nutrition to an enteral feeding program. Cancer Res., 47, 3309-3316.

Torosian, M.H., Tsou, K.C., Daly, J.M., Mullen, J.L., Stein, T.P., Miller, E.E., Buzby, G.P. (1984). Alteration of tumor cell kinetics by pulse total parenteral nutrition. Cancer, 53, 1409-1415.

Valdivieso, M., Frankmann, C., Murphy, W.K., Benjamin, R.S., Barkley, T., McMurtrey, M.J., Jeffries, D.G., Welch, S.R., Bodey, G.P. (1987). Long-term effects of intravenous hyperalimentation administered during intensive chemotherapy for small cell bronchogenic carcinoma. Cancer, 59, 362-369.

Weiner, R.S., Kramer, B.S., Clamon, G.H., Feld, R., Evans, W., Moran, E.M., Blum, R., Weisenthal, L.M., Pee, D., Hoffman, F.A., DeWys, W.D. (1985). Effects of intravenous hyperalimentation during treatment in patients with small-cell lung cancer. J. Clin. Oncol., 3, 949-957.

Long-term Survival and Toxicity in Small Cell Lung Cancer: The Experience of the Umbrian Lung Cancer Group

M. Tonato*, L. Crinò*, S. Darwish*,
B. Biscottini*, P. Latini[+], E. Maranzano[+]
and F. Checcaglini[+]

*Department of Internal Medicine, Regional Hospital,
Terni;
[+]Radiotherapy Unit, Division of Medical Oncology,
Policlinico Perugia, Italy

ABSTRACT

We present the outcome of 99 SCLC patients 4 to 9 years after treatment with
combination chemotherapy with or without chest and cranial irradiation from 1978
through 1983.
Ten patients (10%) all with limited disease survived free of cancer for 30 months
or more and were considered long-term survivors.
Chronic neurotoxicity and pulmonary dysfunction were studied with
neuropsychologic tests, C.T. scan and ventilation tests. Chronic toxicity appears
troublesome, but doesn't outweigh the benefits of prolonged survival and
potential cure.

KEYWORDS

Small cell lung cancer; chemotherapy; long-term survivors.

INTRODUCTION

In the past decade, the prognosis of patients with small cell carcinoma of the
lung (SCLC) has improved by treatment with aggressive combination chemotherapy
and radiotherapy. Currently, 15%-25% of patients with limited disease can be
expected to live beyond two years. These patients are therefore at risk for
manifesting long-term complications that may be related to the treatment.
Many recent reports have indicated a quite variable incidence of such side
effects.

MATERIAL AND METHODS

We have reviewed our experience with 99 SCLC patients treated at our istitutions
between 1979 and 1983 with combined chemotherapy and radiation according to
Livingston's protocol. Staging was performed according to the current accepted
criteria. Limited disease was defined as tumor limited to one hemithorax,
including omolateral, mediastinal and supraclavicular nodes, excluding pleural
involvement.
Of the 99 patients, 53 (53.5%) were limited stage and 46 (46.5%) were extensive
stage. Patient characteristics are reported in table I. All patients received

induction chemotherapy with cyclophosphamide (750 mg/mq), doxorubicin (50 mg/mq), and vincristine (1 mg). CTX and DX were given every 3 weeks, and VCR every week for a total of 12 doses. At the end of the induction period, responding patients were treated with chest and whole-brain irradiation (30 Gy in 10 fractions). After one additional cycle of chemotherapy a boost of 15 Gy was given on tumor volume at the 14th week. Of the patients with extensive disease, only complete responders received prophylactic whole brain irradiation. During radiation therapy only VCR was administered. Combination chemotherapy was resumed at the 12th week and continued with CTX and DX given every month until a total dose of 450 mg/mq of DX was reached. At that point methotrexate was substituted for DX. Chemotherapy was continued a maximum of two years.

TABLE I   PATIENT CHARACTERISTICS

	L.D.	E.D.
n.	53	46
m/f	46/7	44/2
Age (average)	58	57
range	43–73	39–72
P.S.		
80–100	38 (72%)	15 (33%)
40–70	15 (28%)	31 (67%)

RESULTS

Results are shown in table II: of the 53 patients with limited disease, 39 (73.5%) responded (18 C R), while of 46 with extensive disease only 11 responded (24%) (1 C R and 10 P R). Ten patients, all with limited disease, were considered long survivors because they lived 3 years or more from the start of treatment without any evidence of SCLC. Two patients died at 37 and 42 months for a cardiovascular disease probably unrelated to the SCLC or its treatment. No autopsy was performed. An additional patient died at 56 months for liver failure. He was an alcoholic and continued to be a heavy smoker. At his death no clinical sign of SCLC could be detected.

TABLE II   RESULTS

Stage	N. pts	CR	PR	Total	Median S.	L.S.
LD	53	18 (34%)	21 (39%)	39 (73%)	13 m.	10
					p 0.001	
ED	46	1 (2%)	10 (22%)	11 (24%)	7 m.	0
All Stages	99	19 (19%)	31 (31%)	53 (50%)	10	

DISCUSSION

At the time of this evaluation, with a follow up ranging from 3 to 8 years, 7 patients are still alive. One patient experiences quite severe neurological symptoms with memory impairment, coordination abnormalities, intentional tremors and ataxia. A CT of the brain showed a severe grade of atrophy. The same neurological disability has been shown in the patient who died at 42 months for cardiovascular disease and in the other who died at 56 months for liver failure. In this last patient the particular metabolic disease and the toxic condition could have played a role in determining the neurological disability. In the seven long term survivors alive to date, we performed a neuropsycologic evaluation, focusing on mental attention, memory and learning, constructional apraxia and mental status (table III).

TABLE III NEUROLOGIC AND NEUROPSYCHOLOGIC EVALUATION

ATTENTION – Letter cancellation task, Picture cancellation task, Trail Making test A e B, Stroop color words-test

MEMORY and LEARNING – Digit span (Wechsler), Block tapping (Corsi), Visual memory (Rey), 15 words test (Rey), 7/24 test (Barbizet Cany)

CONSTRUCTIONAL APRAXIA – Copying geometrical figures (Arrigoni De Renzi)

INTELLECTUAL FUNCTION – Progressive Matrices C 47 (Raven)

MENTAL STATUS – Orientation to person, place and time, Information memory concentration test (Blessed-Roth)

Memory and learning appear moderately impaired in all the patients, while mental status seems to be in some degree deteriorated in most of them (table IV). However, the quality of life of all the patients didn't worsen along the years of follow-up; they seem to fit quite well in their particular sociofamiliar enviroment and they don't complain of difficulties with relatives and friends in daily life. All of them present a life style common to retired people and are fully able to take care of them selves. C.T. scan of the brain shows ventricular dilatation and atrophy probably in only two cases related to brain irradiation.

CONCLUSIONS

Evaluating the results of neuropsychologic tests, it seems difficult to discriminate between the impairments due to age deterioration and those related to medical treatment.

The relatively low incidence in our series of disabling neurological side effects could be related to the fact that we did not use drugs such as nitrosoureas nor a concomitant radio–chemotherapy with MTX that could adversely affect the neurotoxicity of the treatment.

Moderate pulmonary fibrosis was quite common in our patients, as shown by routine chest x–ray. Five of the 7 surviving patients complain of a certain degree of exertional dyspnea (table V).

No serious hematological disorder has been documented and no second malignancy has developed to date.

Our results are in agreement with what is reported in the literature as regards the percentage of long term survivors in SCLC. Since a late relapse can occur even after 3 years, a careful follow up of these patients is mandatory.

In conclusion, our experience shows that moderately aggressive treatment could determine the same results in SCLC as more aggressive regimens, sparing long term toxicity and without significantly impairing the quality of life of survivors.

REFERENCES

1) N. Ellison, A. Bernath, R. Kane et al. - Disturbing problems of success: Clinical status of long-term survivors of small cell lung cancer (SCLC) - Proc Am Soc Clin Oncol. 1982:C-579.

2) B.E. Johnson, D.C. Ihde, P.A. Bunn et al. - Patients with small cell lung cancer treated with combination chemotherapy with or without irradiation - Ann Int Med. 1985;103:430-438.

3) R.B. Livingston, R.L. Stephens, J.D. Bonnet et al. - Long-term survival and toxicity in small cell lung cancer - Am J Med 1984;77:415-417.

4) J.D. Looper, L.H. Einhorn; S.A. Garcia et al. - Severe neurological problems following successful therapy for small cell lung cancer (SCLC) - Proc Am Soc Clin Oncol. 1984;C-903.

5) H. Scher, B. Hilaris, R. Wittes - Long term follow-up of combined modality therapy in small cell carcinoma (SCLC) - Proc Am Soc Clin Oncol. 1983;C-777.

6) S.A. Volk, R.F. Mansour, D.R. Gandara et al.- Morbidity in long-term survivors of small cell carcinoma of the lung - Cancer 1984;54:25-27.

7) K. Osterlind, H.H. Hansen, P. Dombernowsky et al - Determinants of complete remission induction and maintenance in chemotherapy with or without irradiation of small cell lung cancer. - Cancer Research 1987;47:2733-2736.

TABLE IV   NEUROLOGICAL ABNORMALITIES IN L.S.

P	Age Sex	Symptoms	Attention	Memory and Learning	Constructional Apraxia	Intellectual Function	Mental Status	CT
S.R.	69 m	–	Abnormal (+)	Abnormal (+)	Normal	Normal	Normal	Moderate senile atrophy
A.D.	60 m	–	Abnormal (+++)	Abnormal (+++)	Normal	Abnormal (++)	Abnormal (++)	Severe atrophy
R.M.E.	60 f	–	Normal	Abnormal (+)	Normal	Normal	Abnormal (++)	–
M.N.	65 m	–	Abnormal (++)	Abnormal (+)	Normal	Normal	Abnormal (+)	–
A.D.	50 m	–	Abnormal (+)	Abnormal (++)	Normal	Normal	Normal	–
G.M.	64 m	–	Normal	Abnormal (+)	Normal	Normal	Abnormal (+)	Moderate senile atrophy
P.V.	61 m	Depression	Normal	Abnormal (+)	Normal	Normal	Abnormal (+)	Ventricular dilatation

M. Tonato et al.

TABLE V   PULMONARY DYSFUNCTION IN LONG-TERM SURVIVORS OF S.C.L.C.

P	Age	Symptoms	Chest Roentgenogram	Forced Expiratory Volume/sec. obs. teor. % (1)	Forced vital capacity obs. teor. % (1)	Conclusions
S.R.	68	None	Mild fibrosis of right upper lobe	2.79 (2.64-106%)	3.61 (3.45-104%)	Normal
A.D.	60	None	Fibrosis from left hilum to left upper lobe	2.50 (2.89-86%)	3.62 (3.66-99%)	Small airways obstruction
R.M.E.	60	None	Normal	1.97 (2.01-98%)	2.42 (2.37-102%)	Normal
M.N.	65	None	Previous lobectomy right upper lobe	3 (2.7-109%)	4.2 (3.5-118%)	Mild small airways obstruction
A.D.	50	Dyspnea on exertion	Previous right lobectomy	1.68 (3.16-55%)	2.10 (3.9-54%)	Mild restrictive disease. Chronic pulmonary abscess
G.M.	64	Dyspnea on exertion	Right parame-mediastinal fibrosis with tracheal shift	1.63 (2.29-71%)	1.91 (2.95-65%)	Mild restrictive disease
P.V.	61	Dyspnea on exertion	Volume loss on the right with fibrosis of right hilum	2.05 (2.87-71%)	2.38 (3.66-65%)	Mild restrictive disease

Limited Disease — Small Cell Lung Carcinoma (LD—SCLC) in a Chemosurgical Approach

A. Paccagnella, F. Sartori, A. Brandes,
G. L. Pappagallo, A. Favoretto, F. Calabrò,
F. Rea, V. Chiarion-Sileni, C. Ghiotto,
A. Fornasiero, G. Sotti and M. V. Fiorentino

Oncology Department, U.L.S.S. 21, Padua, Italy

ABSTRACT

From November '82 to January '87, 217 patients (pts) entered our controlled trials. Of the 91 pts with LD, 59 were eligible for the surgical approach; 53 (24%) had resection, 3 eligible pts progressed during induction chemotherapy and became inoperable and in 3 pts no resection was possible at thoracotomy. Staging procedures included brain, chest and upper abdomen CT-scan plus laparoscopy, bone scan, and bone marrow biopsy. Staging mediastinoscopy was carried out in most pts eligible for surgery without overt signs of mediastinal involvement.
The 23 pTNM stage I-II pts underwent surgery followed by chemotherapy (6 courses alternating DXR-VCR-CTX and DDP -VP16 q 21 days) and Prophylactic Cranial Irradiation (PCI).
The 19 pTNM stage III pts received induction CT (4 cycles) followed by Surgery and PCI. Further CT (3 cycles) was given to radically resected pts. Mediastinal radiation was added for pts with tumour in resection margins or nodal involvement.
Eleven additional "clinically" stage I-II pts submitted to initial Surgery, showed mediastinal node involvement being "surgical" stage III; they received chemotherapy as second line treatment. 17/23 (74%) pTNM stage I-II pts and 9/30 (30%) pTNM stage III pts are still alive and disease free with a median follow-up of 34 (10-56) and 16 (6-57) months respectively.
The estimated survival at 3 years is 78% for all pTNM stage I and II and 19% for all pTNM stage III patients.
The chemo-surgical approach induce a considerable number of long term survivors in stage I-II pts. Further follow-up is required to assess the usefulness of surgery in stage III SCLC patients.

KEYWORDS

Small cell Lung Cancer; Limited disease; Surgery in combination with

chemotherapy;   Clinical and Pathological stage correlation; Pattern of relapse;
Multiple and mixed histologies; Survival analysis.

INTRODUCTION

Small cell carcinoma of the lung is usually a sistemic disease at the time of
diagnosis with only one third of cases apparently confined to one hemithorax
and its nodal drainage (Johnson, 1986).
Local treatments with surgery and radiation alone   failed because of occult
distant metastases (Matthews, 1973) (Fox, 1973).
Considerable progress has been achieved in recent years with combination
chemotherapy, complete responses ranging from 20% to 60% with about 20% of long
term survivors in limited stage (Hansen, 1980).
Radiation treatment of the primary in patients obtaining a complete response to
chemotherapy failed to show a survival benefit, patients relapsing within the
hemithorax as well as at distance (Bunn, 1981). In about 30%-40% of cases,
however, the primary site is the only site of disease recurrence or progression
(Hansen, 1980).
This report presents the preliminary results of our prospective study, aiming
to assess the role of surgery in combination with chemotherapy to prevent both
local and distant relapse and to define the relationship between the clinical
TNM staging and the pathological TNM staging as verified at thoracotomy.

MATERIAL AND METHODS

Patients

From November 1982 to January   1987 there were 217 patients seen at Medical
Oncology in Padua with newly diagnosed Small Cell Lung Cancer (SCLC).
All patients had a complete history and physical examination. Pre-therapy
staging included chest X-ray and tomography of the affected   lung and
mediastinum or thoracic CT scan, bronchoscopy and lung function tests, upper
abdomen CT scan or sonography,   laparoscopy with liver biopsies,   CT or
radionuclide brain scan, bone scan and bone marrow aspiration. Most patients
presenting without   overt signs of metastatic dissemination underwent
mediastinoscopy and,   if required,   anterior mediastinotomy.   Alkaline
phosphatase, SGOT, BUN, LDH,   bilirubin, creatinine,   serum electrolytes,
calcium and phosphorus, blood counts were also obtained. Out of 217 patients
with pathologically confirmed SCLC, 126 (58%) had extended disease and 91 (42%)
limited disease (i.e. disease confined to one lung, the mediastinum, and
ipsilateral and/or contralateral supraclavicular lymph nodes). The median age
was 57 years (37 to 73) and the median performance status 70 (40 to 90) on the
Karnofsky scale. There were 196 men and 21 women.

Eligibility

Criteria for eligibility included the following: histologic verification, based
on the W.H.O. criteria, at our centre , performance status of at least 50, age

less than 70 years, no prior malignancy within the previous 5 years excepting for non melanoma skin cancer.

Patients were required to be able to undergo a complete resection of the tumor. No prior therapy except surgery for patients with small peripheral SCLC and without macroscopic signs of mediastinal node involvement requiring a diagnostic thoracotomy was also required.

Patients with   macroscopic evidence of mediastinal node involvement at thoracotomy were operated again and resected after induction chemotherapy. All patients were clinically classified according to the TNM classification (C-TNM) and staged according to the American Joint Committee recommendations for staging .   All operated patients were assigned a pathologic (P TNM) stage. Surgery consisted of resection of the primary tumor and specimens from the bronchopulmonary,   hylar,   subcarinal and paratracheal lymph nodes   for pathologic staging.

Study Design

Clinical stage I and II patients were submitted to surgical resection as initial therapy and then to adjuvant chemotherapy.

Chemotherapy consisted of courses of Doxorubicin (50 mg/m^2), Cyclophosphamide (1200 mg/m^2) and Vincristine (1 mg/m^2) by bolus intravenous injection (CAV) · alternating with courses of Cisplatin (60 mg/m^2) day 1 and Etoposide (120 mg/m^2) days 1, 3 and 5.   Cisplatin was administered over a 2 hour period together with appropriate hydration and forced diuresis. The interval between treatments was 3 weeks and six cycles were delivered.

Clinical stage III patients were submitted to induction chemotherapy with four cycles alternating CAV and Cisplatin plus Etoposide, followed by surgery for non-progressing patients.   Thoracic radiotherapy was added after surgery only for patients with tumor in resection margins or with massive nodal involvement. Radiotherapy consisted of 40 Gy in 20 fractions.

Further 3 cycles of CCNU (75 mg/m^2) orally day 1, Methotrexate (40 mg/m^2) i.m. days 1, 8, 15, 22 and Procarbazine (100 mg/m^2) orally, days 1 through 14 (CMP) was given as consolidation chemotherapy.

Only one among the six patients submitted to thoracic radiotherapy for incompletely resected tumor was able to receive the 3 CMP planned consolidation cycles because of prolonged myelotoxicity (median 1 cycle, range 0-3).

Prophylactic cranial irradiation (17 Gy in 2 fractions) was administered after chemotherapy in clinical stage I and II patients,   and after   surgery in clinical stage III patients.

Patient assessment during and after therapy

Complete blood counts, biochemical profile and interval histories were taken before each cycle of chemotherapy.   Thoracic and upper   abdomen CT scan and fiberoptic bronchoscopy with biopsies were repeated at the end of treatment.

Patients were scheduled for routine follow-up at 3-month intervals for 2 years and   6-month intervals thereafter. Follow-up procedures   included physical examination, chest X-ray, bone and brain scans, liver sonography; biopsies were used to confirm recurrence.

Survival was measured from day 1 of treatment to the date of death or last

follow-up. The analysis included any kind of event including deaths for a
second primary tumor. Survival and remission duration were estimated using the
Kaplan Meier method; differences between curves were analyzed using the log-
rank test.

RESULTS

Fifty-nine out ninety-one (65%) patients with limited disease were eligible for
combined surgery and chemotherapy. They represent the 27% of all patients with
SCLC referred to our centre during the study period. Thirty (51%) patients were
"oat cell carcinoma", 25 (42%) were of intermediate type and 4 (7%) of mixed
histological subtype. Among the 59 eligible patients, 3 with clinical stage
III progressed during induction chemotherapy and became not-candidates for
operation. Two additional patients in clinical stage II and one in clinical
stage III underwent thoracotomy but did not undergo resection because of
extensive mediastinal metastases (Table 1).

TABLE 1 Operability in relation to disease
extension in 217 SCLC patients

	PTS	%
INOPERABLE		
ext	126	58%
lim.	32	15%
OPERABLE (LIM)		
resected	53*	24%
unresectable	6	3%

* 23 (11%) P-TNM stage I and II   and
30 (13%) Stage III

All 59 eligible patients were however included in survival analysis. Among the
53 (24% of all SCLC) resected patients 11 (21%) had a pneumonectomy, 39 (73%)
a lobectomy, and 3 (6%) a segmental resection.

Stage I and II patients: clinical and pathological staging
evaluation

The results of staging evaluation are summarized in Table 2.

TABLE 2   Correlation between clinical
                 and pathologic TNM stage

STAGE		C-TNM PATIENTS		P-TNM PATIENTS	
I	$T_1 N_0 M_0$	7	12%	5	8%
	$T_2 N_0 M_0$	19	33%	14	24%
	$T_1 N_1 M_0$	1	2%	0	___
II	$T_2 N_1 M_0$	9	15%	4	7%
	TOTAL	36	62%	23	38%
III	$T_1 N_2 M_0$	0	___	3	5%
	$T_2 N_2 M_0$	13	22%	21	36%
	$T_3 N_0 M_0$	3	5%	3	5%
	$T_3 N_1 M_0$	2	3%	2	3%
	$T_3 N_2 M_0$	5	8%	7	12%
	TOTAL	23	38%	36	62%

* C-TNM = Clinical TNM;
  P-TNM = Pathologic TNM (at thoracotomy)

Twenty seven patients with clinical stage I, and 9 with clinical stage II (16% of all SCLC patients) underwent initial thoracotomy. Microscopic mediastinal node involvement was found in 8 out 27 (30%) clinical stage I patients and in 3 out 9 (33%) clinical stage II patients. Two additional stage II patients showed unresectable macroscopic mediastinal involvement. Twenty-three (64%) out 36 clinical stage I and II patients were pathologic stage I and II (11% of all SCLC patients). They had a curative resection, received the adjuvant chemotherapy and the PCI.

Out of the 13 clinical stage I and II patients but pathologic stage III, 11 received the same treatment sequence of the pathologic stage I and II patients, and the 2 patients with unresectable disease received chemotherapy only.

The treatment sequences are summarized in Table 3.

TABLE 3   Treatment sequencies

	P-TNM STAGE	PTS	
		RESECTED	UNRESECTED
SURG. + CHEMOTH.	I + II	23	--
	III	11	2
CHEMOTH. + SURG.	III	19	4
TOTAL		53	6

Stage III patients: response to chemotherapy

The 23 clinical stage III patients underwent induction chemotherapy.
Ten patients (43%) obtained a clinical Complete Response and 9 (39%) a Partial response. In 4 patients (18%) there were a stable or progressive disease. All the 19 responding patients had the tumor resection.
One of the 4 non responsive patients was submitted to thoracotomy showing a non resectable tumor.
The correlation between the clinical and pathological responses to chemotherapy for the 20 patients submitted to thoracotomy after the induction chemotherapy is summarized in Table 4.

TABLE 4 Correlation between clinical and pathologic
responses of induction chemotherapy in 23
clinical stage III patients

	CLIN. RESP.		PATHOL.RESP	
	PTS	%	PTS	%
CR	10	(43)	4	(18)
PR	9	(39)	15+	(64)
PROGR.	4	(18)	4*	(18)

+ Microscopic Residual Only
* not eligible for resection, only one evaluated with
   thoracotomy

In 4/10 patients the clinical Complete Response was pathologically confirmed. In partially responding patients residual disease was generally found inside the necrotic tissue: in 6 case in both the primary tumor and lymph nodes, in 7 in the primary only and in 2 cases in lymph nodes only.

Survival Analysis

Seventeen out 23 (74%) p-TNM stage I and II patients are still alive and disease-free with a median follow-up of 34 (10-56) months and with an estimated disease free survival of 67% and an overall survival of 78% at 3-years (Fig.1).

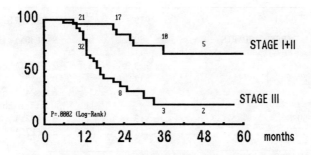

Survival   of   23 pathological   Stage I + II
and   36   pathological   Stage III   patients.

The nodal status (N_1 versus N_0) and the "central" versus "peripheral" site of
tumor origin seem not to influence the outcome of this subset of patients. The
patients with a preoperative diagnosis of SCLC seem to have a disease free
survival similar to that of the patients diagnosed at thoracotomy (Table 5).

TABLE 5 Pathologic stage I + II: disease free patients

	PTS	DISEASE FREE PTS
TOTAL *	23	17 (74%)
N_0	19	14 (74%)
N_1	4	3 (75%)
PRE-SURGICAL DIAGNOSIS	7	5 (71%)
SURGICAL DIAGNOSIS	16	12 (75%)
PERIPHERAL	6	5 (83%)
CENTRAL	15	10 (67%)
FOLLOW-UP more than 24 Mos	18	13 (72%)

* Median Follow-up more than 34 Mos (10-56)

Nine (30%) out 30 patients with P-TNM stage III (23 clinical stage III plus 13
clinical stage I and II but pathologic stage III)   are disease free with a
median follow-up of 16 (6-57)   months. The disease free survival seems not
correlated with the treatment sequences (initial versus post surgical
chemotherapy) and with central versus peripheral site of tumor origin (Tab.6).

TABLE 6   Pathologic Stage III: disease free patients

		PTS	DISEASE FREE PTS
TOTAL * (RESECTED PTS)		30	9 (30%)
N_0		3	3 (100%)
N_1		2	0 (0%)
N_2		25	6 (24%)
CHEM.-SURG.		19	6 (32%)
SURG.-CHEM.		11	3 (27%)
CENTRAL		14	4 (28%)
PERIPHERAL		15	5 (33%)
FOLLOW-UP	more than 12 Mos	27	9 (33%)
FOLLOW-UP	more than 24 Mos	9	3 (33%)

* Median Follow-up 16 Mos (6-57)

Nodal status seems to play an important role since 3 out 3 patients with T3 N0
P-Stage are disease free at 15, 46 and 50 months respectively. Only 7 out 27
(26%) with positive mediastinal nodes are disease free .
Two of the 4 patients showing no microscopical disease in the resection
specimens after induction chemotherapy relapsed locally after 15 and 30 months
and died after 33 and 42 months respectively.
The life table   estimates   for all 36 pathological   stage III   eligible
patients (resected plus   unresected)   show an   overall survival of 19% at 3-
years (median 17 months) significantly   lower than   that (78%) of the 23
P-TNM Stage I+II patients (P = .0002) (Fig. 1).
The survival analisis based on the clinical TNM stage equally show a
significant   survival   advantage   for the 36 C-TNM Stage I + II patients (23
P-TNM Stage I + II plus 13 P-TNM Stage III) over the 23 clinical C-TNM Stage
III patients (19 resected plus 4 unresectable) with a 3 year estimated survival
of 49.6% versus 26.3% (P   =   .0169) (Fig. 2).

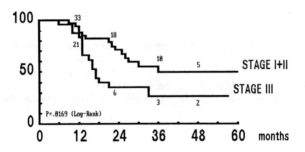

Survival of 36 clinical Stage I + II
and 23 clinical Stage III patients.

Patterns of relapses

Among the 23 P-TNM stage I and II patients, 3 recurred locally. Two patients showed distant metastases only, in both cases to the brain despite prophylactic cranial irradiation. One patients recurred both locally and in distant sites.
Among 36 P-TNM stage III patients, 8 recurred locally, 4 both locally and in distant sites, and 3 at distance only. Two patients died of non-neoplastic disease, one for myocardial infarction and one for pulmonary embolism. At post-mortem examination no tumor persistance was found. In 3 patients having dead for progressing disease it was not possible to assess precisely the sites of recurrence.
Multiple and mixed histology tumors were observed in ten cases (Table 7). Three patients showed head and neck squamous cell cancer: in one of the three cases the secondary tumor was the cause of death after 68 months from resection of Small Cell Lung Cancer.
In 7 cases a double histology was observed inside the lung. Four cases expressed mixed small cell and non-small cell lung cancer, at resection.

TABLE 7   Mixed and multiple cancer

EXTRAPULMONARY (true multiple)		1) LIP SQUAMOUS (previous)
		2) LARINX SQUAMOUS (sincronous)
		3) LARINX SQUAMOUS (subsequent) +
PULMONARY (multiple or mixed)	SINCRONOUS (same lobe)	1) CARCINOID (at diagnosis)
		2) BLASTOMA (after chemotherapy)
		3) ADENOCARCINOMA (after chemotherapy)
		4) SQUAMOUS (at diagnosis)
	SUBSEQUENT (other site)	1) SQUAMOUS (necroscopy) +
		2) SQUAMOUS (contralateral with mediastinal nodes) +
		3) LARGE CELL (second lobectomy)

+ Cause of death

In 3 other cases a second primary of non small cell histology originated in a site distant from that of the resected small cell cancer. In two patients a well differentiated squamous cell carcinoma of the opposite lung was found after 23 and 27 months from the diagnosis of the SCLC. A third patient underwent a right upper lobectomy for a large cell carcinoma after 42 months from initial medial lobe resection for SCLC. The patient is still alive and disease free at 45 months.

DISCUSSION

The role of surgery in the treatment of small cell lung cancer is still controversial. Based on the encouraging results published by Meyer, the present study was designed to evaluate in a controlled setting the proportion of patients eligible for surgery, the proportion of resectable patients, the correlation between the clinical and the pathological TNM stage, as verified with the tumour resection. Despite the lack of randomization, other goals included information on the influence of resection in local control, and survival (Meyer, 1982).

An additional end point was that of testing a third generation combination chemotherapy (CAV alternating with Cisplatin plus VP16) to induce a high proportion of pathologically confirmed complete responses in a selected group of limited disease patients.

The estimates of operability in SCLC are based on retrospective reviews. The majority of the operated patients underwent surgery without a preoperative diagnosis of SCLC.

In a large retrospective analysis by Mountain out of 615 consecutive patients, 3% were resected for an undiagnosed SCLC. In the Shields series 4.7% of the patients underwent the diagnostic resection (Mountain, 1987; Shields, 1982).

In the Osterlind series out of 874 patients, 150 (17%) were retrospectively evaluated as operable. Ninety-six (11%) underwent thoracotomy, 52 (6%) had a radical resection and 54 (6%) were not operated (Osterlind, 1986).

In a prospective study by Williams with surgery as adjuvant after initial chemotherapy, 38 (20%) out 189 patients were eligible for this program. After chemotherapy 13 were considered inoperable, 7 of them because of progression under induction chemotherapy. Twenty-one (11%) patients only were resectable at thoracotomy. It must be pointed out that patients with peripheral localizations diagnosed at thoracotomy were excluded from this protocol (Williams, 1987).

The estimates of operability and resectability from those studies seem to underestimate, for different reasons, the SCLC patients eligible for a surgical approach.

The design of our study based on TNM staging permits to include all SCLC patients operable according to the criteria for non small cell lung cancer.

Since patients with clinical TNM Stage I and II were planned to receive chemotherapy after surgery it was possible to include patients diagnosed not only before surgery but also at surgery . The clinical Stage III operable patients received surgery as an adjuvant to induction chemotherapy. Out of 217 patients, 59 (27%) were eligible for the study and 53 (24%) of them had the resection.

The thoracotomy planned for all our clinical TNM Stage I and II patients permitted to identify the patients with early mediastinal node involvement not otherwise detectable.

About one third (13 out 36) clinical stage I and II patients showed microscopic mediastinal involvement and were pathologic stage III. Even if the treatment sequence was different from that of patients with massive mediastinal node involvement (clinical and pathologic stage III) it seems that the outcome of the two groups is comparable (table 6).

A carefully histological examination of the excised mediastinal lymph nodes seems, therefore, a powerful prognostic tool in operable patients with apparently localized tumor.

The relevance of regional node involvement is again suggested by the outcome of the patients with T_3 N_0 disease since 3 out 3 are disease free at 15, 46, and 50 months (table 6).

Similar results have been observed in T_3 patients by Meyer (Meyer 1985).

Up to now no randomized studies are available to define the uselfulness of surgery in combination with chemotherapy in Small Cell Carcinoma.

Retrospective analyses of series of patients treated with adjuvant chemotherapy after the tumor resection showed different results reflecting different selection criteria.

Shields reported a 5 year survival of 23%. Nine out 10 patients in the Meyer series remained disease free from 6 to 69 months. Maassen reported a survival of 25% with a minimun follow-up of 3 years, Shepherds an estimated 5 year survival of 24%, Friess a 2 year survival of 45%; Davis a two-year survival rate of 39% with a 65.3% for local and a 37.8% survival rate for regional stage cases. (Shields, 1982; Meyer 1982; Maassen, 1985; Sheperds, 1983; Friess, 1985; Davis, 1985).

Osterlind reported a 3 year disease free survival of 33% (12/36) for completely resected patients, of 12.5% (2/16) for resected with residual tumor and 13% (7/54) for operable but not operated patients, including that resection, "per se", had only minor influence on long term survival.

The results we obtained in the subset of patients submitted to adjuvant chemotherapy after initial resection are not directly comparable to those of the quoted studies because of the patients selection based on the TNM staging system we adopted .

As shown by the British Medical Research Council trial, surgery, "per se", is not an effective treatment for Small Cell Lung Cancer. (Fox, 1973).

In a combined modalities treatment setting, however, the results could, at least partially, depend on the characteristics of the adopted combination chemotherapy.

Alternating CAV with Cisplatin- VP16 for 6 cycles as adjuvant to surgery we obtained, in patients with pathologic TNM Stage I and II an estimated disease free survival of 67% at 3-years with 17 out 23 (74%) patients alive and disease free. The estimated survival for the clinical TNM Stage I and II patients (23 P-TNM Stage I and II and 13 P-TNM Stage III) is of 49.6% at 3-years with 20 (56%) out 36 patients disease free (fig. 1). The pathologic stage at initial resection seems to be of prognostic value independently from the possibility to obtain the diagnosis before thoracotomy or at thoracotomy. In our series 5 (71%) out of 7 patients with P-TNM Stages I and II with presurgical diagnoses were disease free as well as 12 (75%) out 16 patient with diagnosis obtained at surgery (Table 5).

Williams recently reviewed the results of five prospective studies planning surgery as adjuvant treatment for limited disease patients responding to combination chemotherapy. Of 69 patients that underwent tumor resection 30 (43%) remained alive and disease free (Williams, 1987).

Baker described a series of 19 patients with limited disease treated with chemotherapy before surgery. Twelve of these patients (63%) are alive and disease free (Baker, 1987).

In our series 6 out 19 patients (32%) treated with the same sequence are alive and disease free with a median follow-up of 16 months (Table 6).

The life table estimates for all the 23 eligible patients (resected plus

140   A. Paccagnella *et al.*

unresectable) showed on overall survival of only 26.3% at 3-years (Fig.2).
Clinical Stage III patients only where, however,   included in this treatment
sequencies.
In only 4 and 10 patients the clinical complete response to chemotherapy,
assessed with CT scan and bronchoscopy was pathologically confirmed.
It is noteworthy that 2 of those patients recurred locally after 15 and 30
months. In the Williams series no one of the 5 patients with no evidence of
tumor in the resected specimens relapsed.
In conclusion, the preliminary data from our study suggest a possible advantage
from the use of surgery combined with chemotherapy.
The benefit seems, however, restricted to the patients with pathologic Stage I
and II.
It seems that operable patients with regional metastases cannot benefit from
this approach, independently from the size of the lymph node involvement and
from the treatment sequencies.
A randomized study is however required to precisely assess the role of surgery
in Small Cell Lung Cancer.

REFERENCES

Baker R.R., D.S. Ettinger, J.D. Ruckdeschel et al., (1987). The role of surgery
    in the management of selected patients with small-cell carcinoma of the lung.
    J. Clin. Oncol., 5, 697-702.
Bunn P.A., D.C. Ihde (1981). Small cell bronchogenic carcinoma: A review of
    therapeutic results. In R.B. Livingstone (Ed.), Lung Cancer, Vol. 1. The
    Hague, Martinus Nijhoff, pp 169-208.
Davis S., P.W. Wright, S.F. Schulman, D. Scholes, D. Thorning, S. Hammer
    (1985). Long-term Survival in Small-Cell Carcinoma of the Lung: A population
    Experience. J. Cl. Oncol., 3, N. 1.
Fox W.,   J.G. Scadding (1973). Medical research Council comparative trial of
    surgery and radiotherapy for primary treatment of small-celled or oat-celled
    carcinoma of the bronchus. Ten year follow-up. Lancet, 2, 63-65.
Friess G.G., J.D. McCracken, M.L. Troxell, et al. (1985). Effect of initial
    resection of small cell carcinoma of the lung: A review of Southwest Oncology
    Group Study 7628. J. Clin. Oncol., 3, 964-968.
Hansen M., H.H. Hansen, P. Dombernowsky (1980). Long-term survival in small
    cell carcinoma of the lung. JAMA, 244, 247-250.
Higgins G.A.   (1972). Use of chemotherapy as an adjunct to surgery for
    bronchogenic carcinoma. Cancer, 30, 1383-1387.
Johnson D.H., F.A. Greco (1986). Small cell carcinoma of the lung. CRC. Crit.
    Rev. Oncol. Hematol., 4, 303-336.
Maassen W., D. Greschuchna, I. Martinez (1985). The role of surgery in the
    treatment of small cell carcinoma of the lung. Recent Results Cancer Res.,
    97, 107-115.
Matthews M.J., S. Kanhouwa, J. Picksen, et al. (1973). Frequency of residual
    and metastatic tumor in patients undergoing curative surgical resection for
    lung cancer. Cancer Chemother. Rep., 4, 63-67.
Mayer J.E. Jr. et al. (1982). Influence of histologic type on survival after
    curative resection for undifferentiated lung cancer. J. Thorac. Cardiovasc.
    Surg., 84, 641-648.

Meyer J.A.,   R.L.   Comis,   S.J.   Ginsberg (1982).   Phase II trial of extended
indications for resection in small cell carcinoma of the lung.   J. Thorac
Cardiovasc. Surg., 83, 12-19.

Meyer J.A., P.M. Ikins, J.J. Gullo, R.L. Comis, W.A. Burke, S.M. Di Fino, and
F.B. Parker (1984). Histologic alterations in small cell carcinoma of the
lung after two cycles of intensive chemotherapy. J. Thorac. Cardiovasc.
Surg., 87, 283-290.

Meyer J.A. (1985).   Effect of histologically verified TNM stage on disease
control in treated small cell carcinoma of the lung. Cancer, 55, 1747-1752.

Mountain C.F. (1987). Operation for Small-Cell Carcinoma Revisited. J. Clin.
Oncol., 5, 687-688.

Osterlind K., M. Hansen, H.H. Hansen, et al. (1985). Treatment policy of
surgery in small cell carcinoma of the lung: Retrospective analysis of a
series of 874 consecutive patients. Thorax, 40, 272-277.

Osterlind K., H.H. Hansen, M. Hansen, et al. (1986). Long-term disease-free
survival in small cell carcinoma of the lung: A study of clinical
determinants. J. Clin. Oncol., 4, 1307-1313.

Osterlind K., M. Hansen, H.H. Hansen, P. Dombernowky (1986). Influence of
surgical resection prior to chemotherapy on the long-term results in small
cell lung cancer: A study of 150 operable patients. J. Clin. Oncol., 5, 589-
593.

Prager R.L., S. Foster, J.D. Hainsworth, et al. (1984). The feasibility of
"adjuvant surgery" in limited stage small cell carcinoma.   A prospective
evaluation. Ann Thorac Surg., 38, 622-626.

Shepherd F.A.,   R.J. Ginsberg,   R. Feld et al. (1983). Reduction in local
recurrence and improved survival in surgically treated patients with small
cell lung cancer. J. Thorac Cardiovasc. Surg., 86, 498-506.

Shields T.W., E.W. Humphrey, C.E. Eastridge, et al. (1977). Adjuvant cancer
chemotherapy after resection of carcinoma of the lung. Cancer, 40, 2057-2062.

Shields T.W., G.A. Higgins, M.J. Matthews, et al. (1982). Surgical resection in
the management of small cell carcinoma of the lung. J. Thorac. Cardiovasc.
Surg., 84, 481-488.

Williams C.J., I. McMillan, R. Lea, et al. (1987). Surgery after initial
chemotherapy for localized small-cell carcinoma. J. Clin. Oncol. 5, 1579-
1588.

Intensification Therapy: High-dose Chemotherapy and Autologous Bone Marrow Transplantation in Small Cell Lung Cancer

M. Marangolo, G. Rosti and M. Leoni

Oncologia Medica, Ospedale Civile, Ravenna, Italy

ABSTRACT

Small Cell Lung Cancer is a tumor higly sensitive to chemotherapeutic agents. Despite this characteristic the duration of disease-free survival is short and the final outcome of patients is very poor: no more than 10-13% of patients achieve long-lasting survival free of disease. Several biological principles are invoked to explain these disappointing end-results: the high growth rate, genetic instability and acquired drug resistance of the minimal residual disease after induction chemotherapy.

High-dose chemotherapy and bone marrow trasplantation as hematological rescue were first adopted in relapsed disease with very poor results. This strategy, however, demonstrated a strict dose - response relationship. For this reason the high dose policy has been employed as a first-line therapy or as late intensification therapy of Complete or Partial Remissions obtained with traditional induction regimens. This strategy seems to be the most promising way to treat Small Cell Lung Cancer.

Sponsored by Istituto Oncologico Romagnolo, grant no. 87232.1

KEYWORDS

High-Dose Chemotherapy; Late Intensification Therapy, Autologous Bone Marrow Transplantation.

Over the past ten years, great effort has been made in improving the cure rate of Small Cell Lung Cancer.
The end-results of chemotherapeutic approaches, 12-40% in terms of Partial or Complete Remissions in the early 1970s, has risen to 60-80% in the recent reports (1,5,20,33).
It is generally agreed that new active drugs and more aggressive chemo-therapeutic regimens are responsible for these interesting results.

The major principles of SCLC therapy drawn from previous experience state
that (1) combination chemotherapy is better than single-agent therapy; (2)
moderately aggressive doses are better than low doses; and (3) tumor shrinkage
occurs quickly during successful therapy.

Although the life expectancy of patients with small cell lung cancer, both
in extended and limited disease, has been prolonged, the cure rate is still
disappointing: no more than 10-13% of patients are alive and free of disease
at 36 months (13, 15).

Several biological properties are invoked to explain the high relapse rate
in spite of the high response rate.

Since the early 1970s, it has become clear that in most patients SCLC is
a disseminated disease at the time of diagnosis; small clusters of cancer
cells may be hiding in biological sanctuaries in which the concentration
of active drugs cannot reach a therapeutic level. These surviving cells
will represent the starting population for a second tumor invasion.

The genetic instability of such a fast-growing tumor increases the probability
of drug resitance to the agent(s) employed as first-line therapy.

Goldie & Coldman's model may justify both the high relapse rate and the
absolute insensitivity to a second-line treatment containing the same drugs
as the induction therapy.

In recent years, several studies have been designed in the light of the
previous considerations reinforced by the excellent results obtained by
the MOPP/ABVD regimen in Hodgkin's Lymphoma. In these studies non-cross-
resistant regimens were alternated over a period of at least 12 months;
this multi-drug attack was supposed to overcome the multi-drug resistance,
thus increasing the cure rate (2,3,6,8,9,10,11,18,19,21,23,32).

Unfortunately the final results of these studies did not confirm the bases
of the rationale. In 717 cases of Limited Disease and 1030 of Extended Disease
treated in 13 trials of alternating chemotherapy from 1979 to 1984, the
median survival was respectively $54+13$ and $35+7$ weeks, in spite of a very
high Complete Remission rate ($46+22$ and $27+10\%$).

Our last reflection on SCLC therapy concerns the low efficacy of second-line
chemotherapies. The poor results of the regimens employed at· relapse are
not only due to the abovementioned biological and pharmacological reasons,
but in part to the poor performance status of relapsed patients; in these
conditions a second-line aggressive chemotherapy is not to be proposed.
It seems, therefore, that various biological aspects cooperate in complicating
the treatment of Small Cell Lung Cancer.

In conclusion, the outcome of patients with SCLC, both in limited and extended
disease, more closely resembles that of patients with Acute Myeloid Leukemia.
The rate of first remission is very high in this disease as well, but the
long-term outcome is very poor and salvage therapies are almost completely
ineffective. The new strategy adopted by Hematologists is to intensify the
complete remission with supralethal chemotherapy and autologous bone marrow
transplantation. This policy has increased the percentage of long-term disease-
free patients, thus obtaining an improvement in the cure rate.

In 1977 it was eperimentally demonstrated by Northon & Simon (22) that small
residual deposits of a tumor highly sensitive to standard chemotherapy,
such as SCLC, can become insensitive to the same drug level. Higher doses
are therefore needed to biologically eradicate them. Hence it seemed reasonable
to employ high dose chemotherapies rescued by Autologous Bone Marrow
Transplantation (ABMT).

The results obtained with high-dose chemotherapy as a salvage   treatment
in relapsed patients have been disappointing. Out of 3 patients previously
treated with combination chemotherapy, Spitzer (28,29) obtained PR lasting
9 months with high-dose BCNU. Out of 9 patients treated with high-dose Cytoxan,
BCNU and VP-16, five PRs and 1 CR with a median duration of 2.5 months were
obtained by the same Author. In both studies the induction chemotherapy
consisted of Vincristine, Iphosphamide, VP-16, Doxorubicin, Methotrexate
and Cytoxan.
With the combination of high-dose BCNU, Procarbazine and L-PAM, Pico (24)
obtained 2 PRs and 2 CRs out of 10 patients, with a response duration of
4 months.
Other Authors treated few patients with second-line therapy consisting of
high-dose chemotherapy and ABMT. Some PRs and CRs were achieved, but the
brief duration of responses reduced the cost-benefit ratio to an unacceptably
low level.
It emerged from these studies, however, that in SCLC the dose-response re
lationship is a rule, even in advanced or relapsed disease. Most patients
did in fact respond again to the same drugs employed in the induction phase
of treatment, when given at a very high dose and rescued by ABMT.
In the light od these data, and considering the high remission rate obtained
by traditional chemotherapy, many Authors have employed high-dose chemotherapy as a front-line in the treatment of SCLC. Interesting results were
obtained by Souhami (27) with Cytoxan 40-50 mg/kg for 4 cinsecutive days
plus Radiotherapy on the chest. In 4 extended and 21 limited disease patients,
4 PRs and 14 CRs were achieved, with a median duration of response of 10.5
months.
Farha (12) treated 14 patients (5 ED, 9 LD) with Vincristine 1.4 mg/sqm
on day 1 plus Cytoxan 1.5 gr/sqm and VP-16 200 mg/sqm for three consecutive
days; 6 PRs and 7 CRs with a duration of 10 months were achieved. Employing
a combination of high-dose VP-16 and Cytoxan (400 mg/sqm and 50 mg/kg
respectively for 2 days) in 18 patients in extended stage, Greco (14) obtained
11 PRs and 5 CRs, with a duration of response of 6 months.
These and other less representative studies can be considered further
confirmation od the principles that (1) SCLC is a sensitive tumor with
a high dose-response relationship, and (2) high-dose chemotherapy should pre-
ferably be given to eradicate small residual disease.
The great majority of trials employing high-dose chemotherapies and Autologous
Bone Marrow Transplantation reserved this modality to late intensification
therapy.
In line with the biological characteristic previously mentioned , and
considering the end results of the high doses in the induction phase, the
treatment of minimal residual disease with supralethal doses rescued by
ABMT seems to be highly rational.
Contradictory results in terms of CRs, duration of responses, and long-term
survival were reported in the first studies, from ca. early 1980 to late
1985 (4,7,16,17,25,31).
Cumulative data from the 6 most representative series show that 190 patients
(50% limited) were treated with induction therapy; late intensification
with high-dose chemotherapy and ABMT were planned, and 129 (67%) completed
the program. The results were quite acceptable: 49 ± 13% CRs, with 27% of
these patients attaining transformed response from PR to CR by means of
high-dose therapies. The median duration of responses was less rewarding,

with a mean value of 34 $\pm$ 9 weeks, and the mean duration of survival increased by 15-50% in comparison with expected results of traditional therapies. In 1986 Spitzer (30) reported the end-results of late intensification therapy in 32 limited-disease patients. After an induction treatment with Vincristine, Iphosphamide and Doxorubicin in 10 patients, or VP-16, Cytoxan, Hydroxydauno-rubicin and Vincristine in 22 patients, all received 2 courses containing high-dose of Cytoxan, VP-16, Vincristine $\pm$ Methotrexate $\pm$ Doxorubicin and ABMT. All patients received radiotherapy of the chest and prophylactic radiaton of the brain.

Complete Remissions increased from 40% after induction therapy to 68% after intensification therapy, the median duration of CRs was 52 weeks and the median survival 92 weeks. These results are quite superior to those previously reported.

Given the biobgical properties of small residual deposits of SCLC, almost 2 consecutive courses of high-doses chemotherapy are probably needed to completely eradicate them. Spitzer's study employed 2 courses of late intensification high-dose therapy and ABMT; this policy, in conjunction with the more active drugs employed, justifies the high cure rate obtained. In 1984 our Group embarked on a pilot study of late intensification therapy in SCLC. Fifteen patients (10 limited and 5 extended) who had achieved CR or PR with Doxorubicin and Etoposide (8 CRs and 7 PRs) were intensified with high-dose VP-16 (1800 mg/sqm in 3 days) and ABMT. After 2 courses of high-dose chemotherapy 11 CRs have been recorded, while 4 patients have remained in PR.

The median disease-free survival is 60 weeks (20-160+) and the overall survival is 70 weeks (52-160+). Four patients are considered long-term survivors and potentially cured, being alive and free of disease at 104, 128, 152 and 160 weeks from the start of therapy. The fifth patient died at 63 weeks without evidence of disease.

This pilot study has demonstrated that high-dose VP-16 and ABMT is a safe single-agent intensification chemotherapy. This policy is probably beneficial in terms of increasing the cure rate of SCLC, but better results can be obtained with a more intensive induction treatment and more aggressive intensification therapy.

REFERENCES

Aisner J., M. Whitacre,D.A Van Echo, and P.H.Wiernik (1982). Combination chemotherapy for small cell carcinoma of the lung: continuous versus alternating non-cross-resistant combinations. Cancer Treat.Rep. 66, 221-230.

Alberto P., W.Berchtold, R.Sonntag, L.Barrelet, F.Jungi, G.Martz, and P.Obrecht (1981). Chemotherapy of small cell carcinoma of the lung: comparison of a cyclic alternative combination with simultaneous combinations of four and seven agents. Eur. J. Cancer Clin. Oncol. 17, 1027-1033.

Aroney R.S., D.R.Bell, W.K.Chan, D.N.Dalley, and J.A.Levi (1982). Alternating non-cross-resistant combination chemotherapy for small cell anaplastic carcinoma of the lung. Cancer 49, 2449-2454.

Banhem S., A.Burnett and R.Stevenson (1982). A pilot study of combination chemotherapy with late dose intensification and autologous bone marrow rescue in small cell bronchoqenic carcinoma. Br. J. Cancer 46, 486-488.

Brower M., D.C.Ihde, A.Johnston- Early, P.A.Bunn Jr., M.H.Cohen, D.N.Carney, R.W.Makuch, M.J.Matthews, and J.D.Minna (1983). Treatment of extensive stage small cell bronchogenic carcinoma: effects of variation in intensity of induction chemotherapy. Am.J.Med. 75, 993-1000.

Cohen M.H., D.C.Ihde, P.A.Bunn, B.E.Fossiek, M.J.Matthews, S.E. Shackney, A.Johnston -Early, A.Makuch, and J.D.Minna (1979). Cyclic alternating combination chemotherapy for small cell bronchogenic carcinoma. Cancer Treat.Rep. 63, 163-170.

Cunningham D., S.W.Banham,A.M.Hutchean,A.Dorward,S.Abmedrai,P.Soukop,DR.Stevenson, R.B.Steck, S.B.Kaye, N.Lucie, A.K.Burnett (1985). High-dose cyclophosphamide and VP 16 as a late dosage intensification therapy for small cell carcinoma of the lung. Cancer Chemoth. Pharmacol.15, 303-306.

Daniels J.R., M.Alexander, M.Kohler, L.Chak, H.J.Lawrence,and M.Friedman (1979). Oat cell carcinoma. Alternating compared with sequential combination chemotherapy. NCOG2061. Proceedings ASCO, 417.

Daniels J.R., L.Y.Chack, B.I.Sikic, M.Mahler, S.K.Carter, R.Reynolds, R.Bohnen, D.Gandara,P.Lockbaun,and J.Yu (1984).Chemotherapy of small-cell carcinoma of the lung: a randomized comparison of alternating and sequential combination chemotherapy programs. J.Clin.Oncol. 2, 1192-1199.

Dombernowsky P., H.H.Hansen, S.Sorenson, and K.Østerlind (1979). Sequential versus non-sequential combination chemotherapy using 6 drugs in advanced small cell carcinoma. A comparative trial including 146 patients. Proceedings AACR 20, 277.

Ettinger D.S., and S.Lagakos (1982). Phase III study of CCNU, Cyclophosphamide, Adriamycin, Vincristine, And VP-16 in small-cell carcinoma of the lung. Cancer 49, 1544-1554.

Farha P., G.Spitzer, and M.Valdivieso (1983). High-dose chemotherapy and autologous bone marrow transplantation for the treatment of small cell lung carcinoma. Cancer 52, 1351-1355.

Ginsberg S.J., R.L.Comis, A.J.Gottlieb, G.B.King, J.Goldberg, K.Zamkoff, A.Elbadawi, and J.A.Meyer (1979). Long-term survivorship in small-cell anaplastic lung carcinoma. Cancer Treat.Rep. 63, 1347-1349.

Greco F.A., D.J.Johnson, K.R.Haude, L.L.Porter, J.D.Heinsworth, and S.N.Wolff (1985). High-dose Etoposide (VP 16) in small cell lung cancer. Seminar in Oncology 12, 42-44.

Hansen M., H.H.Hansen, and P.Dombernowsky (1980). Long term survival in small cell carcinoma of the lung. JAMA 244, 247-250.

Ihde D.C., A.S.Lichter, A.B.Deisseroth, P.A.Bunn, D.N. Carney, M.H.Cohen, R.W.Makuk, A.Johnston-Early,and J.D.Minna (1983). Late intensive combined modality therapy with autologous bone marrow infusion in extensive stage small cell lung cancer. Proceedings ASCO, 198.

Klarstesky J., C.Nicaise, E.Longeval, and P.Strykmaus (1982). Cisplatin, adriamycin, etoposide (CAV) for remission induction of small cell bronchogenic carcinoma. Cancer 50, 652-658.

Krauss S., S.Lowenbraun, A.Bartolucci, R. Buchman, and R.Birch (Southeastern Cancer Study Group) (1981). Alternating non-cross-resistant drug combinations in the treatment of metastatic small cell carcinoma of the lung. Cancer Clin. Trials 4, 147-153.

Livingstone R.B., J.G.Mira, T.T.Chen, M. McGauran, J.P.Costanzi, and M.Sanson (1984). Combined modality treatment of extensive small cell lung cancer: a Southwest Oncology Group study J.Clin.Oncol. 2, 585-590.

Morstyn G., D.C.Ihde, A.S.Lichter, P.A.Bunn, D.N.Carney, E.Glatstein, and J.D.Minna (1984). Small cell lung cancer 1973-1983: early progress and recent obstacles. Int.J.Radiation Oncology Biol.Phys. 10, 515-539.

Murray N., P.Klimo, J.Goldie, E.Hadzic, C.Fryer, N.Voss, and G.Gudauskas, Cancer Control Agency of British Columbia (1982). Alternating combination chemotherapy for small cell carcinoma of the lung (SCLC). Proceedings ASCO, 151.

Norton L., and R.Simon (1977). Tumor size, sensitivity to therapy and design of treatment schedules. Cancer Treat. Rep. 61, 1307-1320.

Østerlind K., S.Sörenson, H.H.Hansen, P.Dombernowsky, F.R.Hirsch, M.Hansen, and M.Rørth (1983). Continuous versus alternating combination chemotherapy for advanced small cell carcinoma of the lung. Cancer Research 43, 6085-6089.

Pico J.L., F.Beaujean, M.Debre, P.Carde, T.Le Cheumbier, and M.Meet (1983). High-dose chemotherapy with autologous bone marrow transplantation in small cell carcioma of the lung. Proceedings ASCO, 206.

Sculier J.P., J.Klarstesky, and P.Stryckmans. (1983). Chimiotérapie intensive tardive avec autogreffe de moelle. Presse Méd. 12, 677-680.

Sikic B.I., L.Y.Chak, and Daniels J.R. (1984). Alternating non-cross resistant chemotherapy of small-cell lung cancer: a controlled trial from the Northern California Group. Inissel BF, Muggia F.M., Carter S.K. (Eds) Etoposide (VP-16) Current status and new development. Academic Press, Orlando, Fla. pp. 197-198.

Souhami R.L., P.G.Harper, D.Linch, C.Tresk, A.M.Goldstone, J.S.Tohies, S.G. Spiro, M.D.Geddes, and J.D.M.Richard (1983). High-dose cyclophosphamide with autologous bone marrow transplantation for the treatment of small cell carcinoma of the bronchus. Cancer Chemoth. Pharmacol. 10, 205-207.

Spitzer G., K.A.Dicke, D.S.Verma, A.Zander, and K.B.McCredie (1979). High-dose BCNU therapy with autologous bone marrow infusion: preliminary observations. Cancer Treat. Rep. 63, 1257-1264.

Spitzer G., K.A.Dicke, and L.Litmen (1980). High-dose combination chemotherapy with autologous bone marrow transplantation in adult solid tumors. Cancer 45, 3075-3085.

Spitzer G., P.Farha, M.Valdivieso, K.Dicke, A.Zander, L.Vellekoop, W.K.Murphy, H.M.Dhingra, T.Umsawasdi, D.Chiuten, and D.T.Carr (1986). High-dose intensification therapy with autologous bone marrow support for limited small-cell bronchogenic carcinoma. J. Clin. Oncol. 4, 4-13.

Steward P., C. D. Buckner, and E. D. Thomas (1983). Intensive chemotherapy with autologous marrow transplantation for small - cell carcinomas of the lung. Cancer Treat. rep. 67, 1055-1059.

Vermorken J.B., J. Stam, N. van Zandwijk, K.J. Roozendaal, J.G. McVie, and H.M.Pinedo (1982). Alternating chemotherapy in small cell lung cancer (SCLC). Proceedings ASCO, 149.

Vogl S.E., and C. Metha (1982). High-dose cyclophosphamide in the induction chemotherapy of small cell lung cancer- minor improvements in the rate of remission & in survival. The III World Conference on Lung Cancer (Abst.), 173.

Second-line Chemotherapy in
Small Cell Lung Cancer

D. Amadori, A. Ravaioli, G. L. Frassineti
and M. P. Innocenti

Department of Oncology, Morgagni-Pierantoni Hospital,
Forlì, Italy

ABSTRACT

Treatment results of small cell lung cancer are still far from satisfactory since
the majority of patients relapse on primary therapy, and thus second line treatments must be developed. Between the prognostic factors affecting the percentages
of the objective response and the duration of the remission in second line therapy, only a limited number has been studied extensively. A good performance status, lack of weight loss, minimal tumor burden, non heavy or cross resistant previous chemotherapeutic regimens, long disease-free interval, no changes in the o-
riginal cytohistological characteristics of the tumor, seem to be favourable prognostic factors. Important biases can be introduced in the evaluation of these
factors by the limited number of patients from each study and by lack of information about patient characteristics. In this review are reported the more effective second line schedules and therapeutic results from the most recent literature
data. From these data the use of Etoposide + Platinum combination as salvage therapy for SCLC in patients pretreated with front line polichemotherapeutic regimens not containing these two drugs seems to be the most effective treatment (CR+
PR: 50%, DMR: 3-5,5 mo., DMS: 3-9 mo. in limited and extended disease).

KEYWORDS

Small cell lung cancer; second line treatments; prognostic factors; therapeutic
results.

INTRODUCTION

The patients who undergo second-line chemotherapy in small cell lung cancer constitute a heterogenous group for several variables. The principle parameters which
define this heterogenicity are as follows: - tumor burden in limited or extended
disease, - aggressiveness and modality of first line treatments, - response to
first line treatments (including response rate, response characteristics and response duration), -morphologic changes in the tumor after intensive chemotherapy.
In order to choose the correct second-line therapy, it is important to take into
consideration the degree of aggressiveness and conditions of first-line treatment.

D. Amadori et al.

FIRST–LINE TREATMENTS: STRATEGY AND RESULTS

Therapeutic strategy in SCLC has developed through numerous approaches, the most important being: chemotherapy with complementary locoregional radiotherapy; the use of non cross–resistant chemotherapy; late intensification chemotherapy; high dose chemotherapy with or without the support of an autologous bone marrow transplantation (ABMT), and chemotherapy with new drugs and new schedules of treatment. At present, scientific discussion regarding first–line therapies is particularly focussed on the following points: – the comparison between the different most effective polichemotherapeutic combinations including Adriamycin, Cyclophospamyde, Vincristine, Etoposide, Cisplatinum combined with or without radiotherapy in the limited and extended stages of the disease; – the role of late intensification chemotherapy, with or without ABMT, after an objective clinical response achieved with induction therapy; – the evaluation of alterning chemotherapeutic non–cross resistant regimens, on the basis of Goldie and Coldman hypotesis; – research into the most appropriate dosage of drugs and the optimal duration of treatments. The results of the principle and most recent studies carried out into this subject are shown in tables 1,2,3.

TABLE 1 Results of First Line Treatments in Limited Stage SCLC

Treatment	N° Pts	CR+PR(%)	CR(%)	MDR (months)	MDS	Ref
CAE–RT+	116	84	47		6–14	2–16–33 43–82
CAEV+–RT	140	84	58		11–21	87–7–83 29–60–19–30
CAEV+–RT vs	175	84	58	12–17(cr)	15	48
CAV+–RT	175	78	55	10–11(cr)	12–14	37
CAE vs	39	64	26	11.5	12	7
CAV	41	56	24	10.5	14.5	
CEV vs	36	61		10.5		13
CAV vs	35	66		10	N.R.	
CV	26	50		11		
EP+–RT	123	91	51		13–22	25–69–41 64–5
CAV/EP + RT	70	93	76	15	19.5	50
CAV/EP + RT vs	152	76	48		15	24
CAV→ EP + RT	145	76	42		15	
	1073					

Longs survivals: 5–10%

The analysis of the above-mentioned studies are as follows: - the various poliche-
miotherapeutic regimens including Antracyclines, Cyclophospamide Etoposide and
Cisplatinum give similar results in terms either of response rate (70–90% with
a CR of 24–76%) or response and survival duration (median values of 10–15 months
and 6–22 months respectively); - the addition of radiotherapy improves the rate
of objective responses however the effect on survival is uncertain.

TABLE 2 Results of First Line Treatments in Extensive Stage SCLC

Treatment	N° Pts	CR+PR(%)	CR(%)	MDR (months)	MDS	Ref.
CAE$^+$RT	154	76	28		6–10	1-2-16-43-49-82
CAEV$^+$ RT	401	81	25		6–12	6-17-7-29-30-45 46-60-80-83-87
CAEV$^+$RT vs	62	84	34	10(cr)	9.5	37
CAV$^+$RT	53	40	14		6.5	
CAE vs	130	54	12	10	10	7
CAV	133	45	10	8	8	
CEV vs	79	48		8		
CAV vs	66	44		7.5	N.R.	13
CV	60	40		6		
EP	163	77	26		9–11	5-25-41-69-78
CAV/EP vs	242	63	40	7.1	9.8	24
CAV		42	27	5.4	7.8	
CAV/HE–E		58	23	11	11.5	21
MTX vs	447					
CAV		59	16	9.7	10	
High Doses	75	81	43	6–10	7.5–11	38-39-72-85
	2075					

Long survivals: ⩽ 2%

Table 2 shows that the most efficacious combinations contain the same drugs as u-
sed in the limited stage; the rate of objective responses is very similar when u-
sing standard and high doses chemotherapy (overall responses not greater than
70–80% with a CR rate of 20–40%). The median duration of response and survival
varies from 5–11 months and 6–12 months respectively with a percentage for long-
term survivors of about 2%.

TABLE 3 Results of Late Intensive (LI) Therapy with ABMT $\overset{+}{-}$ RT in Limited and Extensive Stage SCLC

Author	N° Pts	H.D. Drugs	Stage	Deaths on LI(%)	New CR %	DFS in LI (%)		Ref.
Smith '85	36	C	L/E	3	33	8	1,5 yr	71
Sculier '85	15	CE	L/E	7	42	7	1 yr	68
Stewart '83	10	C	L/E	30	40	10	1 yr	76
Klastersky '82	13	PAE	L/E	15	25	8	1 yr	42
Spitzer '86	32	CE	L	0	47	19	3 yr	74
Humblet '85	19	CEB	L/E	21	86	17	2 yr	34
Banham '85	45	CE	L/E	2	18	4	1.5 yr	3
Cornbleet '84	5	L–PAM	L (cr)	0	–	20	1 yr	14
Ihde '86	8	CE	E	25	20	0	2 yr	35
Marangolo, Amadori '87	15	E	L/E	0	57	27	2 yr	47

(From Ihde '86 Mod.)

The use of Late Intensification treatment gives a new percentage for complete responses of about 40%, which establishes an overall rate for CR of about 75%. The highest percentage of disease-free patients at 3 years is reported by Spitzer in the limited stage of the disease treated with supplementary radiotherapy, and reaches as much as 19%. The reported data show that attempts to develop effective salvage therapy with refractory and resistant tumor are important. Treatment results of small cell lung cancer are still far from satisfactory since the majority of patients relapse on primary therapy and ultimately succumb to their disease (Greco, 1985; Joss, 1986)

SECOND LINE THERAPIES

Response Predictive Factors.
The patients who become candidates for second-line chemotherapy constitute an extremely heterogenous group and the variables for this have been previously reported. As far as concerns the predictive factors of response to second-line chemotherapy, these are closely linked to patient and tumor characteristics and to the characteristics of previous therapy. The major response predictive factors are:
- a good performance status and absence of weight loss; - a minimal tumor burden;
- no changes in the cyto-histological characteristics of the tumor; - the absence of gene amplification (32,40). Prognosis is significantly affected by the characteristics of previous treatments. Patients who have not been heavily pre-treated with multidrug regimens or who have not had cross resistant chemotherapy show a better response to second-line therapy. In addition, a long drug-free interval between first and second-line treatments and slight mielotoxicity from previous treatments enable an adequate dosage of second-line drugs to be administered, which results in an improved therapeutic efficacy. Previously reported studies show that the majority of patients, as a result of the increasing use of multi therapeutic strategies, in particular those employing high drug dosage with or without ABMT, reach second-line therapy with unfavourable prognostic conditions. In addition, in the majority of cases, many of the most efficacious drugs have already been used sequentially or alternately in particularly aggressive first-line regimens. It is little wonder, therefore, that the results obtained up to now are

discouraging using both mono and polichemotherapy.

Result of Second-Line Chemotherapy
The results of second-line monochemotherapy are reported in table 4

TABLE 4 Second Line Monochemiotherapy: Results from 25 Trials

Drug	N° Pts	CR + PR (%)	MDR (months)	Ref.
Etoposide	316	11,5	2,5	36-22-11-77-79
Cisplatin	109	19	3	61-44-8-15
Teniposide	87	17	3,5	53-86-65-28
Vindesine	74	20	3	26-52-81-51
Carboplatin	26	19	4	70
TOTAL	612	85/612 (14%)	2,5-4	

Globally, the results are disappointing, (objective responses from 10–20% with a
low median duration of response)like those obtained with Cisplatin and Etoposide,
while good prospects seem likely from the use of new drugs such as Vindesine and
Carboplatin. Polichemotherapy would seem to have some advantages over monochemotherapy.

TABLE 5 Second Line Polichemotherapy: Results from 16 Trials

Drugs	N° Pts	CR + PR (%)	MDR (months)	MDS	Ref.
VLB-PCB-ADM	13	23	1.5		72
VCR-ADM-PCB	17	59	5.5		12
VDS-CDDP	22	18	6		9
CCNU-VCR-MTX-PCB	29	31	3-7	3-6.5	56
CDDP-VP$_{16}$	210	50	4-5	5,5	20-78-57-62-23-4
High-Dose+ABMT	40	40	2-9		63-58-59-74-55-54-18
	331	148/331 44.7%	1,5-9		

In table 5 are shown the results obtained from 16 trials in second-line polichemotherapy. The objective responses achieved with second-line polichemotherapeutic
combinations range from 20 to 50% with a median response duration of 4-5 months
and overall survival rate of 5 months (8 months in the limited stage). The 7
trials which used high-dose therapy + ABMT did not achieve better results; in fact
objective response rate was of 40% with a median response duration of 2-9 months.
This research was, however, carried out on a limited number of patients with various combinations of drugs, and therefore a more thorough evaluation is necessary. The second-line polichemotherapeutic combination which achieved the best results was that of Cisplatinum and Etoposide (EP) (Table 6)

TABLE 6   Second Line Chemotherapy in SCLC: CDDP + VP_{16} (EP) Results

Author	N° Pts	CR+PR(%)	CR(%)	PR(%)	DMR(months)	DMS	Ref.
Einhorn '84	32	50	9	41	4.7	5.3	20
Tinsley '83	15	47	–	47	N.R.	N.R.	78
Porter '85	29	52	7	45	3	4	57
Rowland '86 + RT	31	71	19	52	N.R.	4	62
Evans '85	78						
– limited	24	63	17	46	5.5	8.75	23
– extended	54	52	4	48	4.5	5.25	
Batist '86	25	12*	–	12	3–4	3	4
	210	106/210 (50.4%)	8%	42%	3–5.5	3–9	

* Patient with negative prognostic factors

Bearing in mind that in monochemotherapy these two drugs have a limited efficacy (a 19% and 11.5% objective response rate for Cisplatinum and VP16 respectively), clinical experience has confirmed a marked synergism in the drugs, as already reported in experimental animal studies carried out by Schabel and Von Hoff at the beginning of the Eighties (66,84). This combination, taking into consideration the entire group of patients suffering from either the limited or extended stage of the disease, produces the following results: – an objective response rate of 50% (12–63%); – a complete response rate of 8% (0–19%); – a median response duration of 3–5,5 months; – a median survival duration of 3–9 months (in both the limited and extended forms of disease). Evans (23) reports different response rates and different characteristics of the response to the EP combination in both limited and extended disease. Table 7 shows the results of second-line chemotherapy, in SCLC with CDDP+VP_{16} (EP)

TABLE 7 Second Line Chemotherapy in SCLC: CDDP+VP_{16} (EP)

Type of response	Disease extent	
	Extensive	Limited
CR + PR	52%	63%
CR	4%	17%
PR	48%	46%
DMR	4,5 mo.	5,5 mo.
DMS		
– overall	5,25 mo.	8,75 mo.
– responders	6,5 mo.	10,5 mo.
– non responders	3,7 mo.	4,5 mo.

Evans 1985

The difference in survival rate between responders and non-responders is not significant. This might depend on the fact that"stable disease" patients, among
whom there was a certain response rate, are included in the non-responders group.
The EP combination, besides having a high therapeutic synergysm, seems, in addition,,to be non cross-resistant with the most widely used chemotherapeutic combination (for example CAV): 47% of non -responders to CAV respond to EP (23).
This likely non cross-resistance is currently being taken advantage of to develop new sequential and alternate approaches to methods of first-line therapy.
On the other hand, little research has been carried out into the possible non
cross-resistance of CAV as second-line therapy compared with the EP combination.
The literature data at present available tend to exclude the bidirectionality of
the non cross-resistance (67). Among the data reported in table 6, Batist's disappointing results (12% overall response; 0% CR; a median response duration
from 3-4 months and a median survival duration of 3 months) are worthy of com-
ment. (4) These differences are probably due to the adverse prognostic factors
which characterize this group of patients: - previous treatment with 6 drugs
(CTX-MTX-CCNU-VCR-ADB-PCB) as compared with 3 drugs used in the other studies;
- long period of drug administration: 7 months versus 5 months (Einhorn, Porter,
Evans); - absence of drug-free interval between first and second-line regimens.
50% of Evan's patients had an interval of roughly 3 months, and all Porter's patients a median interval of 5 months; - low dosage of drugs administered: consequence of high toxicity from initial treatment; - greater possibility of the occurrence of cellular resistant clones with a first-line therapy using 6 drugs
(cross resistance between CMP-VAP vs EP). With respect to survival, the results of
salvage therapies remain, in any case, very disappointing (not more that 4 months
with conventional therapies and not more than 6 months with high-dose therapies).

Toxicity of EP Combination.
The toxicity of the EP combination in second-line treatment results mainly in
mielotoxicity. Porter reports that, out of 88 courses of therapy, only 52 (59%)
could be given at 100% of the planned dose. 15 (25%) out of 59 repeat courses of
treatment met with a delay as a result of myelosuppression which manifested is-
self at nadir levels of 1000 white blood cells per mm^3 and   15.000 platelets
per mm^3 in 35% of patients. Evan's data show slight myelosuppression, above all
with regard to white blood cells. (Only 4% of patients experienced intense toxicity). Slight to moderate hypomagnesaemia, anaemia, nausea and vomiting represent
the other most common toxic side-effects associated with this treatment, which
can also be administered in the out-patients department. All in all the results
of second-line chemotherapy are disappointing and it is therefore necessary to
develop new drug combination and to design new randomized studies to achieve any
further improvement as regards survival and quality of life.

CONCLUSIONS

At present with the most common salvage therapies it is possible to obtain only
a small advantage in terms of survival (not more than 4 months with standard therapies and not more than 6 months with high doses). These disappointing results
of second line chemotherapies underline the need for new developments in salvage
chemotherapy to achieve an improvement in survival and in quality of life. Future
directions for more efficacious second-line therapies can be summarized as follows:
- new multidrug second line combinations, not cross resistant with the first line chemotherapy are needed to be tested either on a clinical or laboratory experi-

mental basis; – identification of new drugs with high degree of activity against
small cell lung cancer must be developed. In table 8 are reportd the new agents
tested in small cell lung cancer in the past few years.

TABLE 8   New Agents in SCLC

Active	Active?
Ifosfamide	Prednimustine
Hexamethylmelamine	Dibromodulcitol
Cisplatin	Iproplatin
Carboplatin	Lonidamine
ACNU	
Vindesine	
Teniposide	

Inactive	Inactive?
Mitomycin	Dianhydrogalactitol
Aziridinylbenzoquinone	HD–Methotrexate
Streptozotocin	PALA
Chlorozotocin	DON
PCNU	Triazinate
5–Fluorouracil	Cytosine–Arabinoside
Vinblastine	Bisantrene
Maytansine	
Amsacrine	
Procarbazine	
Mitoguazone	
Mitoxantrone	
Interferon–	
Zinostatin	
Aclarubicin	
∝–Difluoromethylornithine	

During the past 5 years Ifosfamide, Hexamethylmelamine, Cisplatin, Carboplatin,
Vindesine, Teniposide and ACNU have been shown to be active agents in SCLC, while
preliminary evaluation of Prednimustine, Dibromodulcitol, Iproplatin and Lonida-
mine suggest that these agents may be active (40); – well designed phase II studies with known and new single agent need to be implemented. In fact many present
day phase II studies do not permit a thorough evaluation of the therapeutic efficacy of new drug. This has been confirmed by Cohen, who analysed 97 single agent
phase II trials carried out on 1502 patients.   Important informations regarding
patient characteristics such as prior treatment status, performance status, stage of disease and degree of weight loss were often lacking in pubblications of
phase II trials.   Furthermore, the majority of agents has been inadeguately tested in terms of number of patients or number of studies per drug.   In fact, from
analysis it has emerged that many trials were carried out on heavily pre–treated
patients, which may have misled the potential therapeutic efficacy of the new
drug; – new doses and new schedules of treatment must be developed (high dosages

with or without ABMT, alternate ao sequential   not cross resistant regimens, research into new synergism between drugs); – adeguate laboratory models for the
in vitro and in vivo drug sensitivity studies could be more widely experienced;
preliminary results show that in vitro drug sensitivity testing predict clinical response to initial chemotherapy and suggest that individualized chemotherapy
may have potential therapeutic benefit (Gazdar 1987); – quality of life of the
patients   has be taken into consideration with reference to the cost/benefit ratio in the choice of mono or polichemotherapeutic regimens as second-line treatments. Other promising areas of study include identification of putative growth
factors and production of monoclonal antibodies; it is hoped that this research
will result in improved therapy and survival for SCLC patients also in second line treatment (Greco 1985).

REFERENCES

1) Abeloff, M. D., and others (1981). Intensive induction chemotherapy in 54 pa-
   pients with small cell carcinoma of the lung. Cancer Treat. Rep., 65, 639–646
2) Aisner, J., and others (1983). Doxorubicin, cyclophosphamide, and etoposide
   (ACE) by bolus or continuous infusion for small cell carcinoma of the lung
   (SCLC). Proc. Am. Soc. Clin. Oncol., 2, 196 (abstr.),
3) Banham, S., and others (1985). The role of VP–16 in the treatment of small
   cell lung cancer: studies of the west of Scotland lung cancer. Sem. Oncol.,
   12 suppl. 2, 2–6.
4) Batist, G., and others (1986). Etoposide (VP–16) and cisplatin in previously
   treated small cell lung cancer: clinica trial and vitro correlates. J. Clin.
   Oncol., 4, 982–986.
5) Boni, C., and others (1985). Cisplatinum plus VP–16 chemotherapy as front-line
   treatment in small cell lung cancer. Proc. Am. Soc. Clin. Oncol., 4, 196
   (Abstr. C 765).
6) Brower, M., and others (1983). Treatment of extensive stage small cell bronchogenic carcinoma: Effects of variation in intensity of induction chemotherapy. Am. J. Med., 75, 993–1000.
7) Bunn, P.A. Jr., F.A. Greco, and L. Einhorn (1986). Cyclophosphamide, doxorubicin and etoposide as first line therapy in the treatment of small cell lung
   cancer. Semin. Oncol., 13 – Suppl. 3, 45–46.
8) Cavalli, F., and others (1980). Phase II study with cis–dichloro–diammine-
   platinum (II) in small cell anaplastic bronchogenic carcinoma. Eur. J. Cancer,
   16, 617–621.
9) Chiuten, D.F., and others (1986). Combinations chemotherapy with vindesine
   and cisplatin for refractory small cell bronchogenic carcinoma. Cancer Treat.
   Rep., 70, 795–796.
10) Cohen, E.A., and others (1985). Phase II studies in small cell lung cancer
    (SCLC): an analysis of 97 trials. Proc. Am. Soc. Clin. Oncol., 4, 190 (abstr.)
11) Cohen, M.H., and others (1977). Phase II clinical trial weekly administration
    of VP 16–213 in small cell bronchogenic carcinoma. Cancer Treat. Rep., 61,
    489–490.
12) Cohen, M.H., and others (1977). Combination chemotherapy with vincristine,
    adriamycin and procarbazine in previously treated patients with small cell
    carcinoma. Cancer Treat. Rep., 61, 485–487,
13) Comis, R.L. (1986). Clinical trials of cyclophosphamide, etoposide and vin-
    cristine in the treatments of small cell lung cancer. Semin. Oncol. 13 –
    suppl. 3, 40–44.

14) Cornbleet, M., and others (1984). High dose melphalan as consolidation therapy for good prognosis patients with small cell carcinoma of bronchus.
Proc. Am. Soc. Clin. Oncol., 3, 210 (abstr.).

15) De Jaeger, R., and others (1980). High dose cisplatin with fluid and mannitol-
induced diuresis in advanced lung cancer: a phase II clinical trial of the
E.O.R.T.C. lung cancer working party (Belgium). Cancer Treat. Rep., 64, 1341-
1346.

16) De Marinis, F., and others (1985). Cisplatin, adriamycin, etoposide (PAE) vs
cytoxan, adriamycin, etoposide (CAE) in the chemotherapy (CT) of small cell
lung cancer (SCLC). Cancer Chemother. Pharmacol., 14, S 19.

17) Dillmann, R.O., and others (1982). Extensive disease small carcinoma of the
lung: Trial of non cross resistant chemotherapy and consolidation radiotherapy. Cancer 4, 4, 2003-2008.

18) Dover, D., and others (1981). High dose combined modality therapy and autologous bone marrow transplantation in resistant cancer. Am. J. Med., 71, 973-976.

19) Eagan, R.T., and others (1981). An evaluation of low dose-cisplatin as part of
combined modality therapy of limited small cell cancer. Cancer Clin. Trials,
4, 267-271.

20) Einhorn, L.H., S.D. Williams, and P.J. Loehrer (1984). Platinum and VP 16
chemotherapy for refractory small cell lung cancer. Proc. Am. Assoc. Cancer
Res., 174, 689 (abstr.).

21) Ettinger, D.S., and others (1986). A randomized comparison of conventional chemotherapy with immediate alternation of non cross resistance disease (E.D.)
small cell lung cancer. Proc. Am. Soc. Clin. Oncol. 5, 170 (abstr.).

22) Evans, W.K., and others (1984). VP 16 alone and in combination with cisplatin
in previously treated patients with small cell lung cancer. Cancer, 53, 1461-
1466.

23) Evans, W.K., and others (1985). Etoposide (VP 16) and cisplatin: an effective
treatment for relapse in small cell lung cancer. J. Clin. Oncol., 3, 65-71.

24) Evans, W.K., and others (1986). The use of VP 16 plus cisplatin during induction chemotherapy for small cell lung cancer. Sem. Oncol., 13 - suppl.3,10-16.

25) Evans, W.K., and others (1986). First line therapy with VP 16 and cisplatin
for small cell lung cancer. Sem. Oncol., 13 - suppl. 3, 17-23.

26) Furks, J. Z., and others (1982). A phase II trial of vindesine in patients
with refractory small cell carcinoma of the lung. Am. J. Clin. Oncol., 5
49-52.

27) Gadzar, A.F., and others (1987). Extensive disease small cell lung cancer
(SCLC): a prospective trial of chemotherapy selection base on in vitro drug
sensitivity testing. Proc. International Conference on Small Cell Lung Conference. Ravenna., 165, (abstr.).

28) Giaccone, G., and others (1986). Lung cancer: phase II trials with teniposide
(vm 26). Proc. Am. Soc. Clin. Oncol., 5, 722 (abstr.).

29) Goodman, G.E., and others (1983). Treatment of small cell lung cancer with
VP 16, vincristine, doxorubicin, cyclophosphamide (EVAC), and high dose chest
radiotherapy. J. Clin. Oncol., 1, 483-488.

30) Gracia, J.M., and A. Jimenez (1982). Chemotherapy combination with cyclopha-
mide (CTX), adriamycin (ADM), vincristine (VCR), and VP 16-213 in small cell
carcinoma of the lung (SCLC) Cancer Chemother. Pharmacol., 7, 199-201.

31) Greco, F.A., and others (1985). Chemotherapy of small cell lung cancer. Sem.
Oncol., 12 - suppl. 6, 31-37.

32) Hansen, H.H., and M. Rorth (1985). Lung cancer. In H.M. Pinedo and B.A. Chabner (Ed.), Cancer Chemotherapy, Vol. 7, Elsevier, Amsterdam. Chap. 17, pp. 302–321.

33) Hoth, D., and others (1980). Limited small cell lung carcinoma. Treatment with chemotherapy alone. Proc. Am. Soc. Clin. Oncol., 21, 455 (abstr.).

34) Humblet, Y., and others (1985). Late intensification with autologous bone marrow transplantation for small cell lung cancer: a randomized trial. Proc. Am. Soc. Clin. Oncol., 4, 176.

35) Ihde, D., and others (1986). Late intensive combined modality therapy followed by autologous bone marrow infusion in extensive stage small cell lung cancer. J. Clin. Oncol., 4, 1443-1454

36) Issell, B.F., and others (1985). Multicenter Phase II trial of etoposide in refractory small cell lung cancer. Cancer Treat. Rep., 69, 127-128.

37) Jackson, D.V. Jr., and L.D. Case (1986). Small cell lung cancer: a 10 year perspective. Semin. Oncol. 13- suppl. 3, 63-74.

38) Johnson, D.H., and others (1985) Extensive stage small cell bronchogenic carcinoma: Intensive induction chemotherapy with high dose cyclophosphamide plus high dose etoposide. J. Clin. Oncol., 3, 170-175.

39) Johnson, D.H., and others (1986). High dose pilot studies in extensive stage small cell lung cancer. Semin. Oncol., 13 suppl. 3, 37-39.

40) Joss, R.A., and others (1986). New drugs in small cell lung cancer. Cancer Treat. Rev., 13, 157-176.

41) Kim, P.N., and D.B. Mc Donald (1982). The combination of VP 16-213 and cisplatinum in the treatment of small cell carcinoma of lung. Proc. Am. Soc. Clin. Oncol., 1, 141 (abstr.).

42) Klastersky, J., and others (1982). Cisplatin, adriamycin and etoposide for remission induction of small cell bronchogenic carcinoma: evaluation of efficacy and toxicity and pilot study of a "late intensification" with autologous bone marrow rescue. Cancer, 50, 652-658.

43) Klastersky, J., and others (1985). Combination chemotherapy with adriamycin etoposide and cyclophosphamide for small cell carcinoma of the lung. A study by the EORTC Lung Cancer Working Party (Belgium). Cancer, 56, 71-75.

44) Levenson, R., and others (1981). Phase II trial of cisplatin in small cell carcinoma of the lung. Cancer Treat. Rep., 65, 905-907.

45) Lowenbraun, S., and others (1981). Intensive chemotherapy in small cell lung carcinoma (SCLC). Proc. Am. Clin. Oncol., 22, 504 (abstr.).

46) Lowenbraun, S., and others (1984). Combination chemotherapy in small cell lung carcinoma: A randomized study of two intensive regimens. Cancer, 54, 2344-2355.

47) Marangolo, M., and others (1987). High dose VP 16 and autologous bone marrow transplantation (ABMT) as intensification therapy of small cell lung cancer (SCLC). A pilot study. Proc. Am. Soc. Clin. Oncol., 6, 180 (abstr.).

48) Marsche, R., and others (1986). Randomized trial of CAV with or without VP 16 for limited disease small cell lung cancer (SCC). Proc. Am. Soc. Clin. Oncol., 5, 669 (abstr.).

49) Matelski, H.W., and others (1984), Adriamycin, cyclophosphamide and etoposide (VP 16 - 213) in extensive stage small cell lung cancer. Am. J. Clin. Oncol., 7, 729-732.

50) Murray, N., and others (1986). Alternating chemotherapy and toracic radiotherapy with concurrent cisplatin-etoposide for limited stage small cell carcinoma of the lung. Semin. Oncol., 13- suppl. 3, 24-30.

51) Natale, R.B., and others (1981). Phase II trial of vindesine in patients with small cell lung carcinoma. Cancer Treat. Rep., 65, 129–131.

52) Osterlind, K., and others (1981). Vindesine in the treatment of small cell anaplastic carcinoma. Cancer Treat. Rep., 65, 245–248.

53) Pedersen, A.G., and others (1984). Phase II study of teniposide in small cell carcinoma of the lung. Cancer Treat. Rep., 68, 1289–1291.

54) Phillipps, G.L. and others (1983). Intensive 1,3 bis (2) chloroethyl-1-nitro-souree (BCNU), NSC n. 4, 366, 650 and cryopreserved ABMT for refractory cancer. A phase I–II study. Cancer, 52, 1792.

55) Pico, J.L., and others (1983). High dose chemotherapy (HDC) with autologous bone marrow transplantation (ABMT) in small cell carcinoma of the lung(SCCL) in relapse. Proc. Am. Soc. Clin. Oncol., 2, 206.

56) Poplin, E.A., and others (1982). CCNU, vincristine, methotrexate and procarbazine treatment of relapsed small cell lung carcinoma. Cancer Treat. Rep., 66 1557–1559.

57) Porter, L.L.,III, and others (1985). Cisplatin and etoposide combination chemotherapy for refractory small cell carcinoma of the lung. Cancer Treat. Rep. 69, 479–481.

58) Postmus, P.E., and others (1984). Cyclophosphamide and VP 16 – 213 with autologous bone marrow transplantation. A dose escalation study. Eur. J. Cancer. Clin. Oncol., 20, 777–782.

59) Postmus, P.E., and others (1985). High dose cyclophosphamide and high dose VP 16 – 213 for recurrent or refractory small cell lung cancer. A phase II study. Eur. J. Cancer Clin. Oncol., 21, 1467–1470.

60) Rome, L.S., and others (1985). Cyclophosphamide, adriamycin, vincristine (CAV) vs cyclophosphamide, adriamycin, vincristine alternating with VP 16 (Etoposide) CAV/E) in the treatment of small cell cancer (SCC) ot the lung. Proc. Am. Soc. Clin. Oncol., 4, 191 (abstr.).

61) Rosenfelt, F.P., and others (1981). Phase II evaluation of cis-diamminedichloroplatinum in small cell carcinoma of the lung. Proc. Am. Soc. Clin. Oncol., 21, 449 (abstr).

62) Rowland, K., and others (1986). Continuous infusion VP 16, bolus cisplatin, and simultaneous radiation therapy as salvage therapy in small cell bronchogenic carcinoma. Proc. Am. Soc. Clin. Oncol., 5, 710 (abstr.).

63) Rushing, D.A., and others (1984). High dose BCNU and autologous bone marrow reinfusion in the treatment of refractory or relapsed small cell carcinoma of the lung. Proc. Am. Soc. Clin. Oncol., 3, 217 (abstr.).

64) Salvati, F., L. Mugnaini, and A.R. Cruciani (1985). Cisplatin and etoposide followed by Adriamycin and cytoxan for treatment of SCLC limited disease. Proc. IV Th World Conference on lung cancer, 7 523 (abst.).

65) Samson, M.K., and others (1978). VM 26: a clinical study in advanced cancer of the lung and ovary. Eur. J. Cancer, 14, 1395–1399.

66) Schabel, F.M., and others (1979). Cisdichlorodiammine platinum (II): combination chemotherapy and cross-resistance studies with tumours of mice. Cancer Treat. Rep., 63, 1459–1473.

67) Scher, H., and others (1985). Intensive induction chemotherapy with cisplatin + etoposide with radiotherapy for small cell lung cancer. Proc. IV th World Conference on lung cancer, 95, 483 (abstr.).

68) Sculier, J.P., and others (1985). Late intensification in small cell lung cancer: a phase I study high doses of cyclophosphamide and etoposide with autologous bone marrow transplantation. J. Clin. Oncol., 3, 184–191.

69) Sierocki, J.S., and others (1979). Cis diamminedichloroplatinum (II) and VP 16-213: an active induction regimen for small cell carcinoma of the lung. Cancer Treat. Rep., 63, 1593-1597

70) Smith, I.E., and B.D. Evans (1985). Carboplatin (JM 8) as a single agent in combination in the treatment of small cell lung cancer. Cancer Treat. Rev., 12 73-75

71) Smith, I.E., and others (1985). High-dose cyclophosphamide with autologous bone marrow rescue after conventional chemotherapy in the treatment of small cell lung carcinoma. Cancer Chemother. Pharmacol., 14, 120-124

72) Sorenson, S., H.H. Hansen, and P. Dombernowsky (1976). Phase II study of vinblastine, adryamycin and procarbazine in small cell carcinoma of the lung. Cancer Treat. Rep., 60, 1263-1266

73) Souhami, R.L., and others (1985). High dose cyclophosphamide in small cell carcinoma of the lung. J. Clin. Oncol. 3, 958-963

74) Spitzer, G., and others (1980). High dose combination chemotherapy with autologous bone marrow transplantation in adult solid tumor. Cancer, 45, 3075-3085

75) Spitzer, G., and others (1986). High-dose intensification therapy with autologous bone marrow support for limited small cell bronchogenic carcinoma. J. Clin. Oncol., 4, 4-13

76) Stewart, P., and others (1983). Intensive chemoradiotherapy with autologous marrow transplantation for small cell carcinoma of the lung. Cancer Treat. Rep., 67, 1055-1059

77) Tinsley, R., and others (1983): Potential clinical synergy observed in the treatment of small cell lung cancer (SCLC) with cisplatin (P) and VP 16-213 (V). Proc. Am. Soc. Clin. Oncol.,198 C-772

78) Tinsley, R., and others (1983): Potential clinical synergy observed in the treatment of small cell lung cancer (SCLC) with cisplatin (P) and VP 16-213 (V). Proc. Am. Soc. Clin. Oncol.,198 C-772

79) Tucker, F.D., and others (1978). Chemotherapy of small cell carcinoma of the lung with VP 16-213. Cancer, 41, 1710-1714

80) Valdivieso, M., and others (1984). Effects of intensive induction chemotherapy for extensive-disease small cell bronchogenic carcinoma in protected environment-prophylactic antibiotic units. Am. J. Med., 76, 405-412

81) Vogelzang, N.J., and others (1982). Vindesine in bronchogenic carcinoma. A phase II trial. Am. J. Clin. Oncol., 5, 41-44

82) Vogl, S., P. Bonomi, and A. Chang (1984). Etoposide (VP-16) in very high doses in combination for small cell bronchogenic carcinoma (SCBC) with moderate doses of adriamycin (A) and cyclophosphamide (C): modest results. Proc. Am. Assoc. Cancer Res., 25, 177 (abstr.)

83) Von Eyben, F.E., and others (1982). Vincristine, adryamycin, cyclophosphamide, and etoposide (VP 16-213) in small cell anaplastic carcinoma of the lung. Cancer Chemother. Pharmacol., 7, 195-197

84) Von Hoff, D.D., and D. Elson (1980). Clinical results with cisplatin in lung cancer. In A.W. Prestayko, S. Crooke, S.K. Carter (Ed.), Cisplatin, Current Status and New Developments, Vol. 1. Orlando, Fla, Academic pp. 445-458

85) Wolff, S.N., and others (1983). High dose etoposide as single agent chemotherapy for small cell carcinoma of the lung. Cancer Treat. Rep., 67, 957-958

86) Woods, R.L., and others (1979). Treatment of small cell bronchogenic carcinoma with VM-26. Cancer Treat. Rep. 63, 2011-2013

87) Zekan, P., and others (1985). VP-16 enhancement of treatment results in extensive small cell cancer of the lung. A randomized trial of the Piedmont Oncology Association. Proc. Am. Soc. Clin. Oncol., 4, 192

Therapeutic Approaches to Small Cell Lung Cancer

R. Livingston

Division of Oncology, Department of Medicine,
University of Washington School of Medicine, Seattle,
Washington, USA

ABSTRACT

Attempts to improve chemotherapy have involved several themes: 1) administration of continued "maintenance" at lower doses after initial induction of response; 2) alternating drug regimens; 3) anticoagulant and antiplatelet drugs; 4) dose intensification; and 5) new agents. Maintenance chemotherapy has been largely discarded. Alternating drug regimens and anticoagulant approaches have yet to demonstrate consistent benefit, but are still under investigation. "Late intensification" chemotherapy appears to be of benefit for limited stage patients and for complete responders with extensive disease. Neither cisplatin nor VP-16 appears to offer real benefit when simply added to a standard regimen, but the combination of cisplatin-VP-16 is highly active and somewhat non-cross-resistant with other induction programs. Very high dose chemotherapy, as induction or consolidation, has promise but remains investigational.

Combined modality approaches with radiation added to chemotherapy have produced inconsistent results, but the best survival outcome appears to result from simultaneous use of chest irradiation and chemotherapy for patients with limited disease. Surgical resection of the primary tumor will probably prove of real benefit in a small subgroup of patients with stage I and II disease.

KEYWORDS

Small cell lung cancer; maintenance chemotherapy; alternating drug regimens; anticoagulant and antiplatelet drugs; dose response hypothesis; late intensification; combined modality therapy.

INTRODUCTION

The first theme to address in a discussion of current therapeutic strategy is properly that of how we may improve the results from chemotherapy, since most patients with small cell lung cancer (SCLC) will die with widely disseminated disease. Several topics in this regard have been vigorously pursued in the past decade and will be briefly reviewed.

© 1988 Pergamon Press plc
Printed in Great Britain

AB-72—L

MAINTENANCE CHEMOTHERAPY

First, let us examine the results of randomized trials involving maintenance chemotherapy, by which I mean that one continues to give repeated courses of treatment, usually at lower doses, of drugs after the induction period is completed and the patient has achieved a remission. Maurer and co-workers (1980) reported, in a study by the Cancer and Leukemia Group B, that there was some survival benefit for patients with limited stage disease who received continued maintenance therapy. This was, however, without a significant effect in time to disease progression. In 1984, Woods reported an Australian trial which failed to show any benefit for maintenance with "CAV" (cyclophosphamide, adriamycin and vincristine) after induction therapy with cisplatin and VP-16. Cullen (1986) recently reported a British trial that demonstrated significant, but modest effects on disease-free and overall survival, confined however to patients with extensive stage disease. Splinter and McVie compared "CAE" (cyclo- phosphamide, adriamycin and etoposide, or VP-16) for 5 vs. 12 courses, in a study for the EORTC. At this meeting, I learned from Dr. Splinter (1987) that the most recent update of this study fails to demonstrate any significant dif- ference between 5 and 12 courses.

My conclusions at this point about maintenance chemotherapy are that there is no consistent evidence of benefit. Today, it is not a part of most investigational programs.

THE USE OF ALTERNATING DRUG REGIMENS

With respect to alternating combinations, the most popular regimen tested as an "alternative" is cisplatin plus VP-16. Several randomized trials have tested this concept with that combination. Feld (1985) reported the results of a Canadian trial in limited stage disease which did not show an advantage for "CAV" alternated with cisplatin-VP-16 compared to the simple administration of repeated courses of CAV alone. Goodman (1986) reported a similar, negative result last year in a study from the Southwest Oncology Group, in which alter- nation of cisplatin-VP-16 with CAV plus etoposide (CAVE) was not superior to repeated administration of the single program, CAVE. Evans (1986) reported a Canadian trial in 1986 with a design very similar to that reported by Feld, but examining patients with extensive rather than limited stage disease: they observed a significant benefit for the alternating approach on disease-free, but not on overall survival. Finally, my Italian colleague, Dr. Boni (1987) pre- sented at this meeting the results of a randomized trial which actually demon- strates superiority for the repeated administration of cisplatin-VP-16, compared to a program in which this regimen was rotated with programs employing other drugs.

There is no consistent evidence of benefit to date from the use of alternating drug combinations. However, investigation continues. It is possible that by altering the timing of chest irradiation in limited disease, or the sequence and timing of the combinations employed, better results may yet be achieved with the regimens presently available.

ANTICOAGULANT AND ANTIPLATELET DRUGS

Next we shall consider the results of randomized trials that look at the value of anticoagulant or antiplatelet drugs added to "cytotoxic" chemotherapy, based on the hypothesis that concurrent inhibition of the metastatic process might result, and be synergistic with the effects of the applied chemotherapy. There was an early, small negative trial reported by Stanford (1979) from Britain, and an early, small positive trial by Zacharski (1981) from the United States, both involving the addition of warfarin (Coumadin) to standard chemotherapy. The

Zacharski trial led to a large, cooperative group study in the US, reported by Chahinian (1985). I recently learned from him that the reported results of that trial lead to the same conclusion as reported then: that the addition of warfarin to a combination called "MACC" (methotrexate, adriamycin, CCNU and cyclophosphamide) resulted in a higher response rate and an early effect on survival in patients with extensive stage disease. By one year, this survival effect had disappeared. Dr. Chahinian's group, the CALGB, is now exploring the addition of warfarin in a randomized trial for limited stage patients. Finally, Lebeau (1986) from France reported last year a randomized trial in which "CCA" (cyclophosphamide, CCNU and adriamycin) plus VP-16 was tested with or without the addition of aspirin as an antiplatelet drug. No benefit from the use of aspirin could be demonstrated.

It seems tentatively appropriate to conclude that, in the absence of a consistent, persistent survival effect, the toxicity of warfarin addition is not warranted. (There have been hemorrhagic episodes, occasionally fatal, reported in all series). Aspirin addition appears to be of no benefit. Interest is now shifting to the use of other non-cytotoxic "adjuvants" with a different rationale, such as phosphodiesterase inhibitors and calcium antagonists.

NEW AGENTS AND COMBINATIONS

In reviewing the topic of new agents let us consider the randomized trials of the added value for incorporation of VP-16 (the most active new agent identified in this disease in the past decade) into the standard regimens. A trial reported by Messeih (1987) showed a higher response rate, but no survival benefit, for the addition of VP-16 to CAV, vs. use of CAV alone. Similarly, Zekan and colleagues (1985) reported a higher response rate, but no survival benefit. In a trial reported by Lowenbraun (1984) for the Southeastern Group (US), CAV was intentionally given at equitoxic doses in a comparison to the combination of CAV plus VP-16: again, no benefit was seen when VP-16 was added.

There have also been a number of randomized trials that involve new drug combinations. My colleagues and I (Livingston, 1986) designed a regimen of combined alkylating agents, based on persuasive preclinical evidence of synergism for such an approach in a variety of animal model systems. However, this "BTOC" regimen showed no advantage over standard CAV. Alberto (1981) from Switzerland was unable to demonstrate benefit from 7 drugs given at once, compared to a more standard 4-drug program. Recently, O'Bryan (1987) in the Southwest Oncology Group, looking at the combination of cisplatin-VP-16 in the salvage setting (after patients had developed disease progression), was able to show a statistically significant survival benefit from this regimen, compared in a randomized fashion to BTOC, in fully ambulatory patients. These results also appear superior to any of our previous results with "salvage" chemotherapy.

In conclusion, the simple addition of an active new agent (VP-16) has been identified as the first "salvage" regimen with effects on survival, implying a clinically measurable degree of non-cross-resistance. Of the available newer agents, carboplatin is under evaluation, as a potentially more efficacious agent than cisplatin (Jacobs, 1987; Smith, 1987).

DOSE INTENSIFICATION

Next we will review the results of randomized trials involving the "dose response" hypothesis, which can be stated simply as "more is better", within the limits of patient tolerance. A small, early trial reported by Cohen (1977) from the NCI (US) indicated an advantage for escalation of drug doses in the "CMC" combination (cyclophosphamide, methotrexate, CCNU). This led to a large, confirmatory trial by the Eastern Cooperative Oncology Group, reported by Vogl

(1982), in which a statistically significant impact on <u>survival</u> in patients with
limited disease was demonstrated from escalation of the agent Cytoxan (cyclophosphamide). A second approach to dose escalation involves its use after the
induction period, or "late intensification". In 1984, my colleagues and I (Livingston, 1984) reported survival benefit for late intensification in <u>extensive</u>
stage patients who had achieved a complete remission with their initial therapy.
We used a late intensification program identical to that used for induction.
Greco (1986, 1987) from the Southeastern Group reported previously and at this
meeting significant survival benefit from late intensification in <u>limited</u> stage
patients, using a different regimen (cisplatin-VP-16) from that employed for
induction (CAV). All of these randomized trials involved relatively <u>modest</u>
increments in drug dosage, possible on an outpatient therapy basis.

A further extension of the dose–response concept is exemplified in certain non-
randomized, phase II trials, in which doses of Cytoxan alone were given which
necessitate an inpatient approach, both for drug administration and for subsequent supportive care (Ettinger, 1978; Souhami, 1985). Response rates have
ranged from 70 to 88%, with complete response rates reported by Souhami (1985)
from England of 44 to 50%, using the highest doses. It should be noted that
autologous bone marrow transfusion support, although it was used in one of these
trials, is now known to be unnecessary for full and rapid hematologic recovery
after doses as high as 200 mg/kg, given over 4 days.

In 1986, the Vanderbilt group from the US (Johnson) reported an approach which
probably represents the ultimate possible intensity for an induction chemotherapy regimen <u>without</u> the use of autologous marrow support. They gave Cytoxan at
50 mg/kg/day for 2 days, VP-16 at 400 mg/m^2/day for 3 days, and cisplatin at 40
mg/m^2/day for 3 days. After two cycles of this "maximal" induction, patients
received 4 cycles of "standard" CAV. This study was confined to patients with
<u>extensive</u> stage disease, and the response rates are the highest yet reported in
that setting: 16 of 18 responded with 12 of 18 complete responses (CR). However, the median duration of the responses was only 8 months. This represents a
very modest improvement over the expected results with more standard doses, and
suggests that simply intensifying induction will not lead to a major improvement
in extensive disease outcome.

One may, however, gain a substantial advantage from the use of ultra-high-dose
"late intensification", especially in the setting of limited stage disease. An
interesting trial along these lines was reported by Humblet and co-workers
(1985), with a recent update provided for me by him at this meeting. After
initial induction with standard doses of CAV plus methotrexate, followed by
cisplatin-VP-16, responding patients were <u>randomized</u> to additional therapy at
standard doses, or to the following late intensification program: Cytoxan 1.5
gm/m^2/day for 4 days, BCNU at 300 mg/m^2, and VP-16 at 125 mg/m^2/day for 4 days,
followed by infusion of stored, autologous bone marrow.

The results of that trial demonstrated that disease-free survival, measured from
the time of <u>randomization,</u> was superior for late intensification. The overall
survival in limited stage patients was also superior for late intensification,
but did not reach statistical significance. Impressively, 7 of 11 limited disease partial responders prior to randomization converted to complete response
after intensification, a result almost unique for the use of delayed chemotherapy.

However, most of the patients entered in this trial suffered from relapse of
their disease, especially at the primary tumor site, and it may be important
that <u>no</u> local therapy, such as radiation or surgery, was employed in the trial.

My own conclusions about dose response are as follows: 1) beneficial effects
are evident for cyclophosphamide, at moderate increments in limited stage disease; 2) "late intensification" is effective and will become a common approach –

it is uncertain whether administration of a "non-cross-resistant" regimen is better; and 3) approaches requiring inpatient supportive care, with or without infusion of the autologous marrow, remain experimental.

COMBINED MODALITIES

I would like now to turn to the second theme which influences our therapeutic strategy in this disease: the use of combined modalities. We can first review the results of randomized trials in which chemotherapy alone has been compared to chemotherapy with chest irradiation added, for patients with limited disease. In a trial reported by Perez (1984) for the Southeastern Group, a tripartite, "split" course of chest irradiation, "sandwiched" between cycles of chemotherapy, produced a significant impact on disease-free survival, but a marginal effect on overall survival. Glatstein and Ihde (1985) from NCI (US) compared CMC alone to that combination with concurrent, shrinking field radiotherapy. In the final analysis of that study, in press with Bunn as the senior author, there is a statistically significant advantage, albeit with considerably more toxicity, for the combined modality approach, both for disease-free and for overall survival. Perry (1987) for the CALGB compared CEV (Cytoxan, etoposide and vincristine) alone to CEV followed by irradiation, and to the simultaneous combination of CEV and irradiation. In 1984, preliminary analysis did not show a difference, but the final analysis of this study does demonstrate a survival advantage for the combined modality approaches over chemotherapy alone. Souhami and co-workers (1984) failed to demonstrate such an advantage for their sequential, combined modality approach vs. chemotherapy alone with AV-CM (adriamycin-vincristine/Cytoxan-methotrexate). Similarly, Greco and colleagues (1986) could not demonstrate an effect from the concurrent addition of a short, split-course radiotherapy program to CAV induction. Finally, Kies (1987) from the Southwest Oncology Group compared CAV alone to CAV followed by chest irradiation in patients who had achieved an initial complete response to induction chemotherapy. The Southwest Oncology Group could demonstrate no beneficial effect from sequenced combined modalities. This led us to abandon the "traditional" sequential approach in the Southwest Oncology Group, and the results reported by Glatstein and Ihde with concurrent combined modalities stimulated us to initiate a groupwide, phase II trial, reported elsewhere (McCracken, 1987) at this meeting by Dr. Janaki (1987). Patients with limited disease received concurrent cisplatin-VP-16 plus vincristine and continuous, fractionated chest irradiation to a total dose of 4500 cGy in 5 weeks (180 cGy per fraction), as well as elective, whole brain irradiation. After 3 induction cycles, chemotherapy was continued with other active drugs according to an alternating scheme.

The results of that trial, in the most recent actuarial projection, demonstrate 40% of all patients entered to be alive at 2 years and show an apparent survival plateau at 35%. This exceeds the results of our 2 previous studies, with 20% survival at 2 years and a plateau at 10%.

To summarize: of 7 randomized trials, 3 demonstrated benefit from added chest irradiation, and this includes 2 of 3 with concurrent chemoradiotherapy. In addition, the most recent completed Southwest Group trial, though non-randomized, involves large numbers of patients and seems to show a survival advantage for concurrent use of chest and brain irradiation with cisplatin and VP-16.

What about the use of surgery in a combined modality approach? For patients with TNM stages I and II small cell lung cancer, uncontrolled data suggest that initial surgical resection, followed by chemotherapy with or without brain irradiation, produces results superior to a "historical control" of surgery or radiation alone. Unfortunately, this presentation is rare; at most, only 5 to 10% of patients with small cell will present with stage I or II disease. Thus, an international controlled trial, such as that currently chaired by Dr. Karrer, will be necessary to answer therapeutic questions in these patients. The role of adjunctive chest irradiation in these patients deserves evaluation. For patients with stage 3 disease (limited), these observations about the role of cytoreductive surgery are pertinent: 1) one randomized trial of its value is in progress, sponsored by the Lung Cancer Study Group; 2) uncontrolled experience suggests little or no benefit to patients with N_2, and possible benefit for stage $T_3N_0M_0$ at presentation; and 3) non-small cell histology and benign histology are common findings in chemotherapy responders subjected to resections (Meyer, 1982; Valdiviesco, 1987).

Some new developments are worthy of mention. The prospective use of in vitro predictive assay to select agents for initial or subsequent therapy is the subject of other speakers at this conference (Carney, 1987; Gazdar, 1987). Chemopotentiation ("making old drugs better") is a topic of great current interest, and may involve electron-affinic "sensitizers" such as SR-2508, modulators of drug resistance such as calmodulin antagonists, or the use of a new and potentially better schedule, such as the divided dose cisplatin reported by our German colleagues (Wilke, 1987).

Monoclonal antibodies may be used for therapy, either alone as in the current NCI (US) trial of bombesin, or conjugated to potential "warheads" such as immunotoxins, radioemitters, or chemotherapy drugs. Finally, biologic response modifiers are of interest. For example, in vitro exposure to interferons may modulate antigenicity and result in augmentation of a host immune response; modifiers of the helper-suppressor cell ratio may have similar value; and interleukin-2, alone or combined with infused effector cells, may be directly cytotoxic.

CONCLUSIONS

In summary, I would suggest these as promising strategies in small cell lung cancer for randomized trials: 1) for chemotherapy, the use of dose escalation for alkylating agents, with emphasis on "late intensification"; 2) for combined modalities, the continued exploration of simultaneous chest irradiation and chemotherapy, with emphasis on specific chemotherapy regimes and variations in radiation fractionation schemes.

Our own current direction in limited disease is shown by a currently active pilot study in the Southwest Group, chaired by Dr. Gary Goodman. It involves concurrent chest irradiation, brain irradiation, and 2 cycles of cisplatin-VP-16 for induction followed by 2 cycles of consolidation chemotherapy using active, but non-alkylator drugs, and a final course of high-dose Cytoxan (50 mg/kg/day for 3 days) as late intensification. We have demonstrated feasibility for this approach and hope to compare it soon to the same program without late intensification in a randomized trial.

These are my concluding observations: 1) curative potential in 10% of limited stage patients may improve to 20-30% with currently available approaches; but 2) increased curative potential for extensive stage patients will require successful new developments.

REFERENCES

Alberto, P., W. Berchtold, R. Sonntag, L. Barrelet, F. Jungi, G. Martz, and P. Obrecht (1981). Chemotherapy of small cell carcinoma of the lung: comparison of a cyclic alternative combination with simultaneous combinations of four and seven agents. Eur. J. Cancer Clin. Oncol., 17(9), 1027-1033.
Boni, C., G. Cocconi, G. Bisagni, G. Ceci, A. Cuomo, and G. Peracchia (1987). The cisplatinum (P) and etoposide (E) combination vs the rotation of three continuation chemotherapy regimens (PE, CAV, CCVM) in small cell carcinoma of

the lung (SCCL). A prospective randomized study. Program and Abstracts, International Conference on Small Cell Lung Cancer, Ravenna, (Italy). p. 173.

Bunn, P. (1987). Manuscript in press. Ann. Intern. Med.

Carney, D. N. (1987). The biology of lung cancer. Program and Abstracts, International Conference on Small Cell Lung Cancer, Ravenna, (Italy). p. 35.

Chahinian, A. P., J. H. Ware, and B. Zimmer (1985). Update on anticoagulation with warfarin and on alternating chemotherapy in extensive small cell carcinoma of the lung. Proc. Am. Soc. Clin. Oncol., 4, 191.

Cohen, M. H., P. J. Creaven, B. E. Fossieck, L. E. Broder, O. S. Selawry, and A. V. Johnston (1977). Intensive chemotherapy of small cell bronchogenic carcinoma. Cancer Treat. Rep., 61, 349-354.

Cullen, M., D. Morgan, and W. Gregory (1986). Maintenance chemotherapy for anaplastic small cell carcinoma of the bronchus: a randomised, controlled trial. Cancer Chemother. Pharmacol., 17, 157-60.

Ettinger, D. S., J. E. Karp, and M. D. Abeloff (1978). Intermittent high-dose cyclophosphamide chemotherapy for small cell carcinoma of the lung. Cancer Treat. Rep., 62, 413-424.

Evans, W. K., N. Murray, and R. Feld (1986). Canadian multicenter randomized trial comparing standard and alternating combination chemotherapy in extensive small cell lung cancer. Proc. Am. Soc. Clin. Oncol., 5, 169.

Feld, R., W. K. Evans, P. Coy, I. Hodson, A. S. MacDonald, and D. Osoba (1985). Canadian multicentre randomized trail comparing sequential and alternating administration of two non-cross resistant chemotherapy combinations in patients with limited small cell carcinoma of the lung. Proc. Am. Soc. Clin. Oncol., 4, 177.

Gazdar, A. F., E. Russell, H. Oie, S. Steinberg, B. Ghosh, R. I. Linnoila, J. D. Minna, and D. C. Ihde (1987). Extensive disease small cell lung cancer (SCLC): a prospective trial of chemotherapy selection based on in vitro drug sensitivity testing (DST). Program and Abstracts, International Conference on Small Cell Lung Cancer, Ravenna, (Italy). p. 161.

Glatstein E., D. Ihde, P. Bunn, A. Lichter, M. Cohen, R. Makuch, D. Carney, and J. Minna (1985). Radiotherapy in management of limited small cell lung carcinoma: a randomized prospective study. Cancer Treat. Symp., 2, 97-100.

Goodman, G. E., and J. Blasko (1986). Alternating chemotherapy with VP-16/cisplatinum and vincristine/adriamycin/cyclophosphamide in limited small cell lung cancer: a SWOG study. Proc. Am. Soc. Clin. Oncol., 5, 169.

Greco, F. A., C. Perez, and L. H. Einhorn (1986). Combination chemotherapy with or without concurrent thoracic radiotherapy in limited-stage small cell lung cancer: a phase III trial of the Southeastern Cancer Group. Proc. Am. Soc. Clin. Oncol., 5, 178.

Greco, F. A., L. Einhorn, D. H. Johnson, and R. Birch (1987). Cisplatin plus VP-16 (PVP_{16}) consolidation following induction chemotherapy with cyclophosphamide, adriamycin and vincristine (CAV) in limited small cell lung cancer (SCLC): a Southeastern Cancer Study Group (SECSG) random prospective study. Program and Abstracts, International Conference on Small Cell Lung Cancer, Ravenna, (Italy). p. 169.

Humblet, Y., M. Symann, and A. Bosly (1985). Late intensification with autologous bone marrow transplantation for small cell lung cancer: a randomized trial. Proc. Am. Soc. Clin. Oncol., 4, 176.

Jacobs, R. H., J. D. Bitran, M. Deutsch, P. C. Hoffman, J. Sinkule, S. Purl, and H. M. Golomb (1987). Phase II study of carboplatin in previously untreated patients with metastatic small cell lung cancer. Cancer Treat. Rep., 71, 311-312.

Janaki, L. M., J. D. McCracken, S. B. Taylor, P. G. S. Giri, G. B. Weiss, W. Gordon, Jr., R. B. Vance, and J. Crowley (1987). Improved response rate and median survival with concomitant chemo-radiotherapy in limited small cell carcinoma of the lung: a Southwest Oncology Group study. Program and Abstracts, International Conference on Small Cell Lung Cancer, Ravenna, (Italy). p. 147.

Johnson, D. H., M. J. DeLeo, and K. R. Hande (1986). High-dose cyclophosphamide, etoposide, and cisplatin induction therapy in extensive-stage small cell lung cancer. Proc. Am Soc. Clin. Oncol., 5, 178.

Kies, M. S., J. G. Mira, J. J. Crowley, T. T. Chen, R. Pazdur, P. N. Grozea, S.
E. Rivkin, C. A. Coltman, Jr., J. H. Ward, and R. B. Livingston (1987). Multi-
modal therapy for limited small-cell lung cancer: a randomized study of
induction combination chemotherapy with or without thoracic radiation in
complete responders; and with wide-field versus reduced-field radiation in
partial responders: a Southwest Oncology Group study. J. Clin. Oncol., 5,
592–600.

Lebeau, B. E., C. L. Chastang, and the "Small Cells" French Group (1986). Small
cell lung cancer: first results of a double-randomized clinical trial on
aspirin and on 6 vs 12 chemotherapy cycles for complete responders. Cancer
Chemother. Pharmacol., 18, (supplement 1), A42.

Livingston, R. B., J. G. Mira, T. T. Chen, M. McGavran, J. J. Costanzi, and M.
Samson (1984). Combined modality treatment of extensive small cell lung cancer: a Southwest Oncology Group study. J. Clin. Oncol., 2, 585–590.

Livingston, R. B., S. Schulman, J. G. Mira, G. Harker, S. Vogel, C. A. Coltman,
Jr., S. E. Rivkin, G. T. Budd, M. R. Grever, and J. Crowley (1986). Combined
alkylators and multiple-site irradiation for extensive small cell lung cancer:
a Southwest Oncology Group study. Cancer Treat. Rep., 70, 1395–1401.

Lowenbraun, S., R. Birch, and R. Buchanan (1984). Combination chemotherapy in
small cell lung carcinoma. Cancer, 54, 2344–2350.

Maurer, L. H., M. Tulloh, and R. B. Weiss (1980). A randomized combined modality
trial in small cell carcinoma of the lung. Cancer, 45, 30–39.

McCracken, J. D., L. M. Janaki, S. A. Taylor, S. P. Giri, G. B. Weiss, and W.
Gordan, Jr. (1985). Concurrent chemoradiotherapy for limited small cell car-
cinoma of the lung. In J. Ishigami (Ed.), Recent Advances in Chemotherapy,
Proceedings of the 14th International Congress of Chemotherapy, Kyoto, 1985,
University of Tokyo Press, Tokyo. pp. 1138–1139.

Messeih, A., J. M. Schwietzer, and A. Lipton (1987). The addition of etoposide
to cyclophosphamide, adriamycin and vincristine for remission induction and
survival in patients with small cell lung cancer. Cancer Treat. Rep., 71, 61–
66.

Meyer, J. A., R. L. Comis, and S. J. Ginsberg (1982). Phase II trial of
extended indications for resection in small cell carcinoma of the lung. J
Thorac. Cardiovasc. Surg., 83, 12–19.

O'Bryan, R. for the Southwest Oncology Group, (1987). Unpublished data.

Perez, C. A., L. Einhorn, and R. K. Oldham (1984). Randomized trial of radiotherapy to the thorax in limited small-cell carcinoma of the lung treated with
multi-agent chemotherapy and elective brain irradiation: a preliminary report.
J. Clin. Oncol., 2, 1200–1208.

Perry, M. C., W. L. Eaton, K. J. Propert, J. H. Ware, B. Zimmer, A. P. Chahinian, A. Skarin, R. W. Carey, H. Kreisman, C. Faulkner, R. Comis, and M. R.
Green (1987). Chemotherapy with or without radiation therapy in limited small-
cell carcinoma of the lung. N. Engl. J. Med., 316, 912–918.

Smith I.E., B. D. Evans, M. E. Gore, V. L. Repetto, J. R. Yarnold, and H. T.
Ford (1987). Carboplatin (Paraplatin; JM8) and etoposide (VP-16) as first-
line combination therapy for small-cell lung cancer. J. Clin. Oncol., 5, 185–
189.

Souhami, R. (1984). Radiotherapy in small cell cancer of the lung treated with
combination chemotherapy: a controlled trial. Br. Med. J., 288, 1643.

Souhami, R. L., G. Finn, and W. M. Gregory (1985). High-dose cyclophosphamide
in small-cell carcinoma of the lung. J. Clin. Oncol., 3, 958–963.

Splinter, T. (1987). Personal communication.

Stanford, C. F. (1979). Anticoagulants in the treatment of small cell carcinoma
of the bronchus. Thorax, 34, 113–116.

Valdiviesco, M. (1987). Unpublished data, MD Anderson Hospital.

Vogl, S. E., and C. Mehta (1982). Standard vs. intensive induction chemotherapy
of small cell bronchogenic carcinoma with cyclophosphamide, CCNU and methotrexate, followed by continued CCcM or cyclic maintenance therapy. Proc. Am.
Assoc. Cancer Res., 23, 155.

Wilke, H., W. Achterrath, H.-J. Schmoll, U. Gunzer, P. Presser, and H. Link (1987). Etoposide (VP-16) and split course cisplatin (DDP) as first line treatment in SCLC. Program and Abstracts, International Conference on Small Cell Lung Cancer, Ravenna, (Italy). p. 155.

Woods, R. B., and J. A. Levi (1984). Chemotherapy for small cell lung cancer (SCLC): a randomized study of maintenance therapy with cyclophosphamide, adriamycin, and vincristine (CAV) after remission induction with cis-platinum, VP16-213 and radiotherapy. Proc. Am. Soc. Clin. Oncol., 3, 215.

Zacharski, L. R., W. G. Henderson, and F. R. Rickles (1981). Effect of warfarin on survival in small cell carcinoma of the lung. Veterans Administration Study No 75. JAMA, 245, 831-835.

Zekan, P., D. Jackson, and H. Muss (1985). VP-16 enhancement of treatment results in extensive small cell cancer of the lung - a randomized trial of the Piedmont Oncology Association. Proc. Am. Soc. Clin. Oncol., 4, 192.

Extensive Disease Small Cell Lung Cancer:
A Prospective Trial of Chemotherapy Based on *in vitro* Drug Sensitivity Testing

A. F. Gazdar, E. K. Russell, H. K. Oie,
S. Steinberg, B. Ghosh, R. I. Linnoila,
J. D. Minna and D. C. Ihde

National Cancer Institute, Naval Hospital Bethesda and
Uniformed Services University of the Health Sciences,
Bethesda, MD 20814, USA

ABSTRACT

We devised a clinical protocol for individualized selection of chemotherapy from small cell lung cancer (SCLC) patients based on in vitro drug sensitivity testing (DST). Because SCLC is seldom resected surgicaly, most specimens consisted of biopsy specimens obtained during routine staging procedures. The tumore cells usually had to be selectively amplified in number by culture in defined HITES medium prior to performance of DST. DST was performed by a dye exclusion method (Weisenthal). Patients were treated with standard front line therapy and restaged at 12 weeks. If they were in complete remission (CR) front line therapy was continued. If not, they were switched to the in vitro best regimen (IVBR) if data were available. If DST data were not available, they were switched to a three drug second line therapy. Cell lines could be established (and DST performed) on nearly half of all the patients from whom a tumor containing specimen was obtained. There was an excellent correlation between DST results and the patients´ responses to initial therapy. In addition, there appeared to be a modest therapeutic advantage of the IVBR over the standard second line therapy.

KEYWORDS

Cell culture, drug sensitivity testing, dye exclusion assay, in vitro best regimen.

INTRODUCTION

SCLC usually is responsive to initial chemotherapy. However, most responders eventually develop tumor recurrence. At the time of recurrence or progression, the tumors usually are resistant to further therapy. We devised a protocol based on idividualized selection of chemotherapy. This presentation represents an interim report on our progress.

While individualized cancer chemotherapy based on in vitro testing has been proposed for more that thirty years, relatively few adequately performed clinical studies have been conducted. One of the major technical problems is the ability to adequately test a sufficiently high percentage of tumor samples. The assay most frequently used has been the clonogenic assay as modified by Hamburger and Salmon (1978). this assay has the major advantage of permitting selective growth of tumor cells while preventing stromal

cell growth. In earlier studies performed in our laboratory, Carney and colleagues (1984) demonstrated that less than 25% of tumor containing specimens
from SCLC patients yielded sufficient clones to test even three drugs at a
single concentration.

Another problem with testing SCLC tumors is that the primary tumors are seldom
resected at many medical centers including our own. In vitro testing has to
rely on routine staging procedures to provide the major source of tumor material.
Only a minority of these specimens contain tumor cells. Further, many tumor
containing specimens contain modest numbers of tumor cells surrounded by large
numbers of stomal cells. Before such a specimen can be tested, the tumor
cells have to be selectively amplified in number and stromal cell growth
suppressed.

PROTOCOL DESIGN

We designed a protocol that circumvented these general and specific problems.
We have considerable experience with the selective growth of SCLC tumor specimens
in defined media (Carney and co-workers, 1985). For in vitro testing wer used
a dye exclusion assay (Weisenthal and colleagues, 1983) that usually can be
utilized successfully if sufficient tumor cells are available. Tumor samples
were obtained during initial staging procedures as well as biopsies of easily
accessible lymph node and subantaneous metastases. Because most SCLC patients
require immediate therapy, etoposide (VP-16) and cisplatin were administered
for 12 weeks. In the interim, tumor cell number amplification was attempted
and in vitro testing performed whenever a cell line was established. For the
purposes of this protocol we defined a cell lines as existing whenever sufficient
in vitro amplification of tumor number had occurred to permit sensitivity
testing with multiple drugs. Most of these so called lines became fully established continuous cell lines.

Drug testing was performed using either one hour or continuous exposure to
seven drugs having known clinical activity against SCLC. The drugs were tested
over a 100-fold concentration range. A drug was considered active if tumor
cell survival at the reference concentration was less than 50%. The reference
concetrations were selected by Dr. Larry Weisenthal after testing large numbers
of lung cancer tumor specimens. They included VP-16, cisplatin, adriamycin,
nitrogen mustard (used as a substitute for cyclophosphamide) vincristine,
lomustine (CCNU) and methotrexate.

After receiving first line therapy for 12 weeks, the patients were restaged.
Further therapy, commencing at week 13 , depended on response and availability
of in vitro test data. Complete responders continued VP-16 and cisplatin
therapy. If in vitro drug sensitivity data were availalbe, partial or non-
responders received a three drug 'in vitro best regimen' (IVBR) constructed
from the most active drugs . If data were not available, they were switched
to the standard 'second line' regimen of vincristine, adriamycin and cyclophosphamide (VAC).

PROTOCOL FEASABILITY

To date, 63 patients with extensive stage SCLC have been entered onto protocol.
From these 168 pre-treatment staging and diagnostic specimens were processed by
the laboratory (2·7 specimens/patient). However, only 69 contained tumor (41%).
Most of the positive specimens were received from bone marrow, lymph nodes and
malignant effusions, and were obtained under local anesthesia. General anesthesia
was required for obtaining only five positive specimens, from mediastinum, lung
and rib. These procedures were usually performed for diagnostic purposes.

malignant effusions, and were obtained under local anesthesia. General anesthesia was required for obtaining only five positive specimens, from mediastinum, lung and rib. These procedures were usually performed for diagnostic purposes.

The 69 tumor containing were obtained from 46 patients (73% of patients entered on protocol). From these we established one or more cell lines from 21 patients (46% of patients from whom a tumor containing specimen was received, or 33% of all patients).

PROTOCOL RESULTS

SCLC cell lines obtained from 21 patients were subjected to chemosensitivity testing. The frequency with which each drug was ´active´ (defined as <50% cell survival at the reference concentration) ranged from 57% for VP-16 to 10% for methotrexate. We also analyzed the number of times an individual drug was among the 3 most effective (irrespective of percentage cell kill). The range was 66% for VP-16 and 20% for methotrexate. By both analyses the rank orders were similar. For number of times ´active´, the rank order was VP-16, cisplatin, adriamycin, nitrogen mustard, vincristine, lomustive and methotrexate. The 21 lines demonstrated considerable heterogeneity in their responses to the drugs, and 14 different three drug regimens were selected as the ´in vitro best regimen´ (IVBR).

There was considerable correlation between the in vitro drug sensitivity patterns and the responses of the patients to initial VP-16/cisplatin therapy. In 14/15 (93%) of cell lines from patients with complete or partial responders at 12 weeks had 2 or more ´active´ drugs, and 43/96 (45%) of individual drug assays yielded less than 50% cell survival at the reference concentration. In contrast, none of 4 cell lines from non-responding patients had 2 or more ´active´ drugs, and only 1/25 (4%) of individual drugs demonstrated ´activity´. These differences are highly significant (p<·003).

Of 12 non-responding patients who received IVBR at week 13, 3 (25%) achieved complete remission. In contrast, only 2/25 (8%) of non responding patients who received VAC at week 13 (because IVBR data was not available) achieved complete remission.

DISCUSSION

Our studies demonstrate that clinical protocols for extensive stage SCLC based on in vitro sensitivity testing are feasible. Nearly 50% of tumor containing specimens can be successfully cultured and tested, even though several of these contained relatively few viable tumor cells. However, the protocol is extemely labor intensive, as most of the specimens lack tumor cells. These samples must be processed and cultured until the lack of tumor cells can be confirmed.

Cell lines from untreated SCLC patients demonstrated considerable heterogeneity in their responses to drugs. This heterogeneity is essential for individualized drug selection. Results of drug sensitivity testing are highly correlated with response to initial chemotherapy. Preliminary data suggest that individualized drug selection may have a modest potential for therapeutic benefit.

Our results are encouraging and future studies may be rely on larger tumor samples obtained surgically. this would permit earlier application of IVBR, and perhaps a larger percentage of patients for whom IVBR data were available. Finally, the clinical/laboratory correlations suggest that screens for newer therapeutic agents based on the use of human tumor cell lines are justified.

REFERENCES

Carney, D.N., Gazdar, A.F., Cuttitta, F., and Minna, J.D. (1984). Lung Cancer. 247-261. Mizell and Correa, Verlag Chemice International.

Carney, D.N., Gazdar, A.F., Bepler, G., Guccion, J.G., Marangos, P.J., Moody, T.W., Zweig, M.H., and Minna, J.D. (1985). Cancer Research, 45, 2913-2923.

Hamburger, A.W., and Salmon S.E. (1977), Science, 197, 461-463.

Weisenthal, L.M., Morsden, J.A., Dill, P.L., and Macaluso, C.K. (1983). Cancer Research, 43, 749-757.